Therapy Techniques
Using the Creative Arts

D1560059

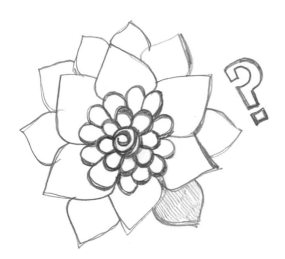

Therapy Techniques Using the Creative Arts

Ann Argé Nathan
Suzanne Mirviss

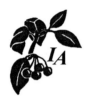

Idyll Arbor, Inc.

PO Box 720, Ravensdale, WA 98051 (425-432-3231)

Cover art by Darrell Nelson
Idyll Arbor, Inc. editor, Denise Juppé

© 1998 Idyll Arbor, Inc.
Second Printing: June 2002

 Idyll Arbor, Inc. supports wise use of our natural resources. This book is printed on recycled paper.

Library of Congress Cataloging-in-Publication Data
Nathan, Ann Argé, 1947-1995.
    Therapy techniques : using the creative arts / Ann Argé Nathan, Suzanne Mirviss.
          p.   cm.
    Includes bibliographical references and index.
    ISBN 1-882883-30-6 (alk. paper)
    1. Arts—Therapeutic use. I. Mirviss, Suzanne, 1950-   . II. Title.
RC489.A72N38 1998
616.89'165—dc21   98-6514
                                                  CIP

ISBN 1-882883-30-6

Acknowledgments

Note from the publisher:

Ann Argé Nathan was a dynamic, warm and caring individual, an exceptional human being who touched the lives of many people. This manuscript was completed with the help of family, friends and colleagues just prior to and after her death. We would like to recognize and thank everyone who generously shared their knowledge, time and skills to complete this book and make it a reality. We have made every effort to include everyone who helped and apologize to anyone whose name we may have inadvertently omitted. Our thanks go to the following people: Reneé Emunah, Arnell Etherington, Lois Herman Friedlander, Betsy Best Martini, Susan Coto McKenna, Charlie Price, Deah Schwartz and Ellie White.

Special thanks go to Ann's family for their help in preparing and completing the manuscript from Ann's notes.

Finally, thanks to Suzanne Mirviss, Ann's teaching partner, who filled in so much of what Ann knew, that Ann didn't have time to put in the book. Without her help this book would have been far less rich in ideas and explanations.

Contents

Acknowledgments..v

1   Introduction..1

2   Elements of Creativity 9

3   Roles of the Therapist 27

4   The Individual and the Therapy Group.....................39

5   Planning for the Creative Arts Group 79

6   Visual and Tactile Arts 103

7   Masks...133

8   An Introduction to Drama Therapy Groups............145

9   Theater Games and Improvisation..........................151

10   Drama...171

11   Laughter and Clowning..193

12   Music..203

13   Dance/Movement and Movement Exploration.....215

14   Poetry and Writing...235

15   Meditation and Creative Visualization 259

References..273

Index 277

List of Activities

Advisor.. 267
Affective Words #1 119
Affective Words #2 119
Alphabet Movement.. 219
Animal Family 128
Animal House 228
Animal Side 123
Animals... 228
Anti-Coloring Book 121
Appreciation Gift 77
As Seen by Others... 129
Association Drawing.. 121
Automatic Drawing... 116
Award... 125
Back Drawing 117
Back Drawing and Writing 245
Back to Back 223
Ball Movement Activities 230
Behind Your Back.. 190
Birthday... 129
Body Parts Game 227
Body Parts to the Floor 225
Body Sculpting in Fours 158
Body Sculpting in Pairs 158
Body Talk... 222
Body Tracing 123
Body Warm Up 217
Bubbles.. 227
Build a Curiosity Picture... 115
Building Together 117
Care Packages for Others.. 127
Circle Form 75
Circle of Love 129
Circle Walk 221
City or Country 168
Clay 115
Clay Exploration (Warm-ups) 112
Closure 222
Clustering/Wandering with Words 251

Collage Messages.. 74
Coloring Book.. 189
Combining Art and Music 109
Complementary Stretching 220
Contact Improvisation... 220
Conversations Between People.. 212
Create a Care Package for Yourself.. 119
Create a Dance 220
Create a Fantasy Creature 112
Create a Me Collage or Me Box 120
Create in Pairs 112
Create the World... 131
Creating a Musical Score 212
Dance Cards 217
Dialogue 244
Diamonte... 256
Double... 191
Drawing Objects Game (a version of Pictionary)............................. 108
Drawing Pass 110
Dream Representation.. 190
Edible Art.. 115
Elbow Tag... 223
Elements.. 130
Eleven Writing Exercises... 243
Empty Chair 188
Essences 147
Events and Emotion 121
Exploration.. 212
Exploration of Trust and Support 219
Eye Contact... 218
Family Crest.. 129
Family Sociogram 128
Finding a Space 225
Finger Painting... 114
Footprints 219
Free Drawings.. 114
Future Projection.. 189
Gift 74
Group Appreciation 75
Group Hug 170
Group Mobile... 129
Group Mural... 109

Haiku 255
Hallucinatory Psychodrama 190
Hand-On-Hand 218
Hero/Heroine 122
Heroic Deed 124
Holiday Memories 250
House, Tree, Person 130
How Do I Feel Now? 119
How Old Am I ? 156
Hula Hoop Activities 230
I Am 249
I Am a Tree 126
I Give You 129
I Remember 252
Images of Self 244
Immediate States of Being 122
Influences 127
Initials 110
Ink Blot 114
Inside/Outside Box 123
Instant Replay 162
Interpersonal Game Rondos 207
Involvement in 3's and 4's 156
Johari Window Exercise 125
Joy/Sadness/World 121
Kinetic Family 128
Laugh It Up 169
Let It All Hang Out 160
Letting Go and Holding On 222
Letting Go of Something 212
Life Line Drawing 125
Line Form 76
Lip Sync 166
Magic Shop 187
Making Captions 253
Masks 124
Medal of Honor 76
Media and Color Exploration 116
Meditation Exercise 260
Message Sending 118
Mirror by the Double 175
Mirror for Expression 191

Mirroring in Groups of Four 220
Mirroring Movement 227
Mirrors 165
More Movement Practice.. 226
Morning Mirror.. 124
Movement Map.. 222
Movement Through 218
Moving to Divergent Emotions 220
Moving to Opposites... 219
Multiple Double 191
Mural... 128
Mural of a Town 110
Music and Markers 254
Name Game Rondos 207
Non-Verbal "Conversation"... 117
Non-Verbal Techniques 189
Observation Game 156
One Day to Relive.. 188
One Wish... 188
One Word Sharing Cards 76
Orientation Game... 155
Our Memory Poem 250
Outright Lie.. 164
Painting Completion 117
Pair Scribble... 116
Pantomime 169
Paper Bag Dramatics... 159
Parachute Activities 232
Passing the Buck 163
Pattern Walk... 227
Pennies Activity 75
Personal Associations/Extensions of Self..................................... 244
Personal.. 148
Personal Shield.. 126
Physical Elevation... 192
Pictionary 117
Picture Mosaic and Enlargement 109
Pictures and Words 247
Play How You Feel and Title It 212
Portraits 127
Positive Lifetime Review.. 125
Positive/Negative Attributes 124

Projective Game Rondos... 210
Projective: Who we are/How we see others 148
Prop Round 159
Props — To Evoke Characters... 244
Radio and TV Exercise — Roving Reporter 159
Rain 212
Real Life Drama... 167
Relaxing the Body... 268
Ripples 166
Road of Life (Picture Autobiography) #1 120
Road of Life (Picture Autobiography) #2 120
Role Reversal in Psychodrama 191
Role Reversal in Role Playing 175
Rondos with Props 209
Scarf Dance 218
Scribble Drawings... 114
Secret Friend 75
Self Book... 122
Self Portrait in Clay 113
Self Portrait on Paper 122
Self Poster 123
Self-Realization.. 189
Sharing Space with Another 130
Show Me How You Feel Game... 161
Small Potato Touch.. 249
Something to Do Together.. 117
Sound and Motion Pass... 217
Statement Completion.. 248
Status Change... 125
Straw Painting.. 115
Sufi Heart Dance 75
Suggesting Movements and Varying Them... 222
Support 127
Symphony of Emotions in Music 161
Symphony of Emotions on Paper 109
Syntu 255
Talk Show 165
The "Land of S" Action Verbs 219
The Human See-Saw... 229
The Three Wizards (also known as "Dr. Know it All") 160
The Where Game 157
Then and Now.. 131

xiii

Think of Someone Who Moves the Way You'd Like To… 221
Three Envelopes 245
Three Wishes #1 119
Three Wishes #2 244
Time Tree 131
Total Group Effort 211
"Touch Blue" Game 228
Toy Talk 252
Transformations 167
Trophy 129
Unfinished Messages 129
Visualization and Affirmation of Forgiveness 266
Visualization Journal 245
Walk My Walk 162
Walking the Line 226
Walking/Moving with Partner 218
Want to Do 120
Watercolor/Crayon Resist 115
Weather Exercise 157
What I Like About Myself 124
Who (or "Who Am I?") Game 164
Who Started the Motion? 163
Who Would You Like to Be? 188
Wish 77
Word Game 158
Word Response 248
Writing Gifts 253
Writing Your Name with an Imaginary Pen 223
You Can Tell How I Feel by the Way that I _____ 221
You'll Never Believe… 246
Your Family 128
Your Future 120
Your World 130
Zen Telegram and Planting Ceremony 246

1

Introduction

...the bulk of psychotherapy is still verbal and still rests on the implicit assumption that the psyche resides in the head and must be approached in the language of the head — words.

— Bernard Feder

This book is an introduction to the process of using the creative arts to help people solve problems and grow. The first part of the book focuses on defining and establishing a basic knowledge of concepts such as:

- creativity and the expression of creativity
- roles that the therapist assumes to enable clients to engage in creative expression
- theories of individual growth and development
- group development and dynamics
- logistics of planning for creative arts groups

The focus of this part of the book is on giving therapists some fundamentals that will help them in leading a creative arts group. It is intended to be practical and applicable and is based on years of experience working with the creative arts in therapeutic and educational settings.

The second section of the book offers creative arts activities that have been used with clients and students. Through the years many students have expressed the idea that leading and participating in these activities impacted the way they viewed themselves both professionally and personally. For students who had been hesitant to lead an arts group, the classroom became a laboratory for trying out and processing the activities. Many realized that they could be successful in using arts activities with groups and wanted to go on to further explore certain creative arts modalities. On a personal level, students experienced what it felt like to participate in the activities themselves and could project what the activities might evoke for clients more realistically. Students became more aware of the value of the creative arts and what it takes to facilitate the activities.

Each creative arts modality chapter consists of (at least) three sections:

- a description of the modality
- considerations for the therapist on running a group with that modality
- activities

There is little debate that the creative arts have an impact on lives, especially the lives of individuals with disabilities. Individuals who struggle with continuous challenges often find great benefits in the experiences that the creative arts offer. These benefits, which can be of value to all individuals, are found in many areas:

- **Expansiveness and freedom.** The creative arts stimulate our senses, our bodies, our thoughts and feelings. For a period of time we are beyond the bounds of time, space and physical limitations. Outside our normal realm of existence, we are free to think, feel and express what seems natural to us.

- **Internal communication.** During creative activity we are linked with our inner selves. We interact with an object or situation and find ways to communicate our thoughts and feelings about what we are seeing or experiencing. While we are involved in creative activity we are engaged in a sustained union with self that is different from normal consciousness and profound because we are closer to touching our unique self.

- **External communication.** When we express our ideas and feelings in a form through the expressive arts, we have the opportunity to say, "This is me. I exist. This is how I feel and see the world." While the sharing of self is often scary for people, it can also create a bridge to other human beings. Those who thought they knew a client well may react with amazement when they observe a piece of artwork that the client has created.

- **Leisure.** During creative activity, it is possible to escape the hectic, overwhelming external and often internal distractions of life. Creative activity freezes time. Many people experience a sensation of "flow" — of being totally engaged and at peace with self during creative activity. Only the activity of that moment exists. We are given the chance to regroup, rethink and reenter the world with a fresh perspective.

- **Alternative communication.** Some creative arts involve expression through images, sound and movement. They bypass left-brain thinking and engage right-brain processing which is more holistic, less detail-oriented, less logical but more integrative. This often enables individuals to explore and express a troublesome thought, feeling or conflict in a new way, through an image, a sound or a movement that communicates it more clearly than ever before. Even when using words, as in a creative writing session, the words have more power and take on an expanded meaning.

- **Self-worth.** The process of expressing creativity involves an exploration of self in order to be able to respond and communicate ideas from a personal perspective. It also involves working materials, words or movements with one's own hands or body and dealing with one's own evaluation of the work and the evaluation of others. This process can be both frightening and joyful. It takes courage to embark on a creative journey in which there are many "what ifs." What if the work doesn't turn out the way I expect it to? What if it's more difficult than I expect it to be? When one still perseveres, witnessing the product of this output of energy is highly validating. No matter how one might feel about the product, an individual can be proud of the journey, of taking a different, unknown path and not turning back.

- **Healing.** The creative arts can be healing in two ways. First, when an individual is deeply involved in the act of creating, s/he may experience a kind of "mental vacation." Individuals who are normally disturbed by thoughts or anxieties will have noticeably more relaxed faces and bodies during creative activity. Relaxation can occur when the chattering, active mind is occupied and thoughts and feelings are channeled into positive activity. Secondly, individuals may experience a surge of energy during creative activity and a feeling of well being. According to Maslow's (1968) hierarchy of needs, the act of creation fulfills the need to explore and express one's potential and validate one's own ability to do more than just survive.

- **Interpersonal relations.** Interpersonal relations are developed through working out problems together. Perhaps the best way to illustrate that creative arts have an impact on how people relate to each other is through the following example: During an art grant project involving veterans with psychiatric disabilities at the VA Medical Center in San Francisco, the group was creating a ceramic tile mosaic panel of an Orca. It required the involvement of many clients to lay out pieces and to glue and grout and it took over two months to complete. During the project, there were some very positive interactions between clients. Individuals were seen trying to help each other problem solve sections of the artwork, assisting in completing sections, taking over responsibility when someone had to leave and giving each other encouragement and praise for completed work. When the group was having a problem getting the mosaic (which weighed over 60 pounds) into the frame, one client who had done carpentry work offered to help and took over leadership to solve the problem. Now the mosaic hangs in the lobby of one of the VA buildings as a testimonial to the beauty that can be created when people work together.

The Art Part and the Therapy Part
(Activity Analysis)

Using the creative arts with clients is really a dual process — one part is carrying out an artistic endeavor and the other part is concerned with understanding how to create an environment which will be therapeutic.

The Art Part
- process
- products
- materials

The Therapy Part
- human development
- group dynamics
- conditions and process of therapeutic change
- personal and professional self-knowledge

In any activity, there is a relationship of parts which can change the nature of the activity. This relationship is illustrated in Figure 1-1, in which areas which may change and have mutual influence appear.

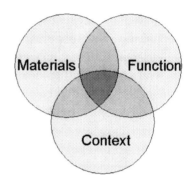

Figure 1-1: Relationship of materials, function and context.

When any of the variables in the diagram alters, it may affect one or both (and sometimes neither) of the others. For example, a game may be played by a group of children as "just a game." It may be played by friends in their leisure time. The function of the game appears to be fun — something to pass the time. If we change the context by playing this game in a therapy session, what else do we change? Perhaps nothing, as we play this game for its own sake. But we could decide to use this game with a group that needs to develop cooperation skills. Now we could add to our list the function of teaching people to work together. The same material is being used but with a new context and function. Context, function and material are variables for the therapist and the group to alter as they wish; this is part of the Activity Analysis Process.

The Arts Are Effective

Because...

Developmentally we learn through doing.

People function on non-verbal as well as verbal levels.

The same defenses and interactions that we create with words are expressed non-verbally with objects.

A creative arts group or experience provides a setting where a microcosm of functioning can be seen.

Art, according to Aristotle, "releases unconscious tensions and purges the soul." It is *cathartic*, that is, the expression of a problem or concern in itself provides relief. This cathartic effect is common to all expressive therapies.

Elements found in the arts, either in individual form or in combination, encourage self-expression and creativity, and bring about enjoyment, insight and knowledge.

Art, as therapist Elinor Ulman (1996) defines it, is "the meeting ground of the world inside and the world outside."

Creative arts therapies maintain that the creative process can be a means of both reconciling emotional conflicts and fostering self-awareness and personal growth. They can provide a careful blend of elements adjusted to the specific needs, personalities and abilities of the individual and the therapist.

2

Elements of Creativity

Every creative act involves...a new innocence of perception, liberated from the cataract of accepted belief.
— Arthur Koestler, *The Sleepwalkers*

As infants we use our senses to learn where we are and who or what is important to our world. Colors and shapes, sounds, taste and touch are the indispensable tools of infancy and childhood. Children have the time to wonder and to gaze with curiosity at everything that crosses their paths, from bugs to stars. The young child creates and imagines, spinning dreams and fantasies and then unraveling them in a second. Adults marvel at these abilities and yet often inadvertently squelch them. As the years progress, natural creativity is often squeezed out by pressures to conform to society's expectations — a society that often values linear thinking and the "right answer" more highly than imagination and lateral thinking. Many adults have the feeling that something is missing in their lives, when the problem is that their abilities to imagine and to create have gone dormant.

This chapter takes a look at the elements of creativity, from the process itself to the personal qualities that foster it, the nature of the "flow experience," and blocks to creativity. It concludes with a list of the conditions that enhance or hinder expression in groups.

✦ What is Creativity? ✦

Creativity is one of those elusive concepts like love and justice that defies definition, though philosophers and artists have been attempting to describe it for centuries. Perhaps one of the most concise definitions comes from Mihaly Csikszentmihalyi (1996), a psychology professor who has extensively researched the topics of flow and creativity. In his book entitled **Creativity**, he writes "Creativity involves the production of novelty." The "ingredients" (ideas, techniques, materials) may be new, or they may be a new combination of existing ingredients, but the product will be something unique to every individual.

The Qualities of the Creative Person

The human qualities that are instrumental to creativity are present in every one of us to some degree. Some individuals are born with physical, cognitive or emotional challenges that make expressing their creativity more difficult. Sometimes circumstances inhibit or damage a person's capacity to experience and express these qualities. Many people in our groups will express the feeling that their creativity has somehow been stifled. For most people this happened sometime in childhood. However, a traumatic event, even in adulthood, can also make it more difficult for a person to risk being creative.

It is one of the tasks of the therapist who uses arts in therapeutic groups to help individuals rediscover their creative selves and validate qualities that spark every aspect of life.

There may be a real set of personality traits by which the naturally creative person can be identified, but this is debatable. There are definitely traits which facilitate the creative process, and it is in the development of these traits that an individual can expand his/her own capacity for being creative. Some traits are very straightforward, but there is a curious aspect that is associated with heightened creativity, and that is the phenomenon of paradoxical traits. These traits involve the ability to move from one extreme to the other as the occasion requires — their development expands the boundaries of the personality. The straightforward traits are

- **Curiosity, wonder and interest**…in what things are like and how they work. Without a good dose of these, it is difficult to recognize an interesting, creative problem.
- **Openness to experience.** A fluid attention that constantly processes events in the environment is a great advantage for recognizing potential novelty.
- **Enjoyment of learning.** Learning brings new information: ideas, thoughts and feelings that can inspire creative endeavors.
- **Tolerance of ambiguity.** Ambiguity has a tendency to make people uncomfortable. But a tolerance for it implies the ability to perceive a greater complexity in the world than our categories sometimes acknowledge and, with that, to enrich the way one sees it. For example, it is possible to mix hundreds or maybe thousands of shades of gray. If the place between black and white is so versatile, why do we keep seeking out the same old colors? Experimenting may produce a gray unlike any other.
- **Risk taking.** Taking risks means accepting challenges that make it necessary to go beyond a certain "personal comfort zone." It means having the courage to stand alone and make a statement. Why take them? Success has its own rewards. But even if a risk fails, the individual has sought out an opportunity to learn new things, to increase his/her comfort zone and tolerance for new experiences. Risk taking enhances self-esteem.

Dialectical

Validation   Challenge

The paradoxical set of traits are arranged as pairs:

- **Playfulness and discipline.** Playfulness is a way of exploring ideas, but after the exploration, it takes perseverance to bring a new idea or vision to completion.

- **Fantasy and realism.** Being creative means alternating between imagination and fantasy at one end and a deeply rooted sense of reality at the other. The individual goes beyond what is considered "real" to create a new "reality." To do this means to be able to clearly perceive the present environment and work with it to produce a new vision.

- **Passion and objectivity.** Creative work demands a passion for the subject on the part of the individual, which motivates him/her to stay with a difficult task, but it also demands an ability to be objective about the flaws and merits of the work, to recognize the real quality of one's work.

Creative Thinking: Left Brain/Right Brain

Collectively, ours is a left-brained culture — one that tends to value thinking that is logical, analytical, verbal and abstract. But humans actually process information in two different ways. Research done over the last 150 years has demonstrated that the left hemisphere of our brains is specialized for language and language functions. The right hemisphere processes information in more holistic (integrated), spatial, intuitive and non-linear ways, seeing "the whole picture" rather than its individual parts. This division is actually something of a generalization — some people (especially left handers) may do verbal information processing in their right hemispheres or in both hemispheres — but by and large the generalization holds — we have two modes for processing information.

What does this mean for creative thinking and how do the two halves of the brain work together? Although the left hemisphere usually dominates (and its functions are most actively developed in schools), sometimes the right hemisphere's mode of information processing is best suited to the task. The left hemisphere analyzes time sequenced events, the right hemisphere synthesizes over space. The brain is task oriented: depending on the nature of the task at hand the hemispheres will work together (each taking on the part of the task that is appropriate to its mode of processing) or singly.

Since the right hemisphere is better at processing many creative arts tasks, the strategy would be to "turn off" the dominant left hemisphere processing and give the reins to the right. But how to do that? One traditional way of silencing the left brain is through meditation. Meditation is a multilevel discipline, but in the initial stages the goal is to "quiet the chattering monkey" (the monkey being the active left hemisphere) so that the person can perceive the world in a more direct and holistic way. In Zen Buddhism the contemplation of a koan, a nonsense question ("What is the sound of one hand clapping?"), brings the student to a greater awareness of reality. The koan can be seen as an attempt to stop logical processing cold by presenting the mind with a completely illogical problem to "solve."

On a more pragmatic level, Betty Edwards (1989) suggests in **Drawing on the Right Side of the Brain** that the way to produce a cognitive shift in processing is to present the dominant hemisphere with a task that it either can't or won't do. She offers a number of drawing tasks that cause the right hemisphere to take over, causing an enhancement in the drawing skills of people who thought that they had no artistic talent.

Those who can effectively utilize both abilities will operate on a more creative level. The process of creation involves both analysis and intuition, words and mental pictures and thought and feeling.

✮ The Creative Process ✮

Creativity can really be thought of as more of a process than a talent or an innate gift. As such it becomes accessible to everyone. It is not just the province of geniuses but is practiced in many forms and by people in a wide variety of disciplines. In a way, it is a form of problem solving, though the problems may be as diverse as expressing a feeling or hypothesizing the structure of DNA.

This process has been explored and written about by countless psychologists and creative people. Traditionally, it is thought to consist of five or six phases (inspiration and preparation are sometimes combined).

1. **Inspiration.** Something in the environment — an issue, a problem, an emotional experience, a landscape — arouses curiosity and interest. There is kind of internal "tension" aroused by the inspiration that needs resolving.

2. **Preparation.** Information gathering. Becoming fully immersed in the "problem." Learning about the topic by observation, researching, talking with other people.

3. **Incubation.** This is what Csikszentmihalyi (1996) calls "the mysterious time." Internal retreat and synthesis. Ideas are churning below the threshold of consciousness, producing unusual and unexpected connections.

4. **Insight.** Sometimes called the "Aha!" experience — when the pieces of the puzzle fall together.

5. **Evaluation.** The phase when a person must decide if an insight is valuable and worth pursuing. This can be an emotionally trying period of self-criticism and insecurity. Is it a novel idea? Will it work? What will others think of it?

6. **Elaboration.** The actual work of creation. This is the hardest work and the most time consuming. Thomas Edison was referring to this phase when he said that creativity was 1% inspiration and 99% perspiration.

Csikszentmihalyi makes the point that in real life there may be several periods of insight, evaluation and elaboration as the person refines his/her work. It is a *recursive* process, one that is repeated over and over again until the person feels that s/he has gotten his/her creation "just right."

Finally, in a creative arts group, there is the period of sharing. Sharing work in which one has invested time and effort can be a delicate business. There is no guarantee that the individual's ideas will be communicated or received exactly as they were intended. This is a vulnerable situation for any creator and especially for our clients. If a time for sharing is set up, there should be ground rules on how feedback is given. There should also be an option *not* to share if a client so chooses. Remind clients always to take what rings true to them and discard what seems like personal taste. If something of value is learned, the individual can note it for future use or return to Phases 5 and 6 of the process.

★Creativity and the Flow Experience★

Ideally, therapists want their clients to enjoy their creative experience. But what is enjoyment? Csikszentmihalyi (1996) studied those who were engaged as professionals in activities that they seemed to enjoy regardless of money or fame. These optimal experiences were often difficult but stretched people's capacities and involved an element of novelty or discovery. He dubbed these "flow experiences." The description of these did not vary much by culture, gender, race or age. According to his research, nine elements describe when an experience is enjoyable:

- **Clear goals.** The person knows exactly what needs to be done next.
- **Immediate feedback to one's actions.** In contrast to everyday life, in a flow experience we know exactly how well we are doing. Each note or brush stroke or move is immediately perceived as right or wrong.

- **A balance between challenges and skills.** If the challenges are too high, people are anxious and frustrated. Too low, and they are bored. In flow, there is the right balance between abilities and challenge.
- **Action and awareness are merged.** In flow, a person's concentration is focused on what s/he is doing, in contrast to ordinary activities, where one may be thinking one thing and doing another.
- **Distractions are excluded from consciousness.** In flow, we are aware of only what is relevant in the here and now. Flow is the result of intense concentration, one that temporarily relieves us of our fears and the cares of everyday life.
- **No worry of failure.** While in flow, the person is too involved to care about failure. Process becomes more important than product.
- **Self-consciousness disappears.** During the flow experience, we are too involved to worry about protecting the ego. Yet after an episode of flow is over, we generally emerge with a stronger self-concept. We have successfully met some challenge. Paradoxically, the self expands through acts of self-forgetfulness.
- **The sense of time becomes distorted.** Generally in flow we forget time. Hours may pass by in what seems like moments. Or time may stretch out — a motion may be fast in clock time, but feel much slower in the time experienced. The sense of time becomes dependent on what we are doing.
- **The activity becomes *autotelic*.** Whenever most of the conditions of flow are present, and as skills increase, an activity begins to become *autotelic*, which is Greek for something that is an end to itself. Many things in life that are done are *exotelic*, not done for themselves but in order to get to some later goal. Some are both. The violinist, for instance, gets paid to do what s/he loves. In many ways the secret to a happy life is to learn to get flow from as many of the activities that we have to do as possible.

It should be apparent that flow experiences are exactly what we are after when we describe the benefits of engaging in creative arts experiences. Yet people are not always ready or willing to engage in creative experiences; they may be blocked or fearful. In order to help people to break out of these self-imposed limits, it is necessary to understand exactly what blocks their creativity. The next section addresses this issue.

★ Blocks to Creativity ★

Why aren't people more creative? In **A Whack on the Side of the Head** Roger von Oech (1993), a successful business consultant in creative thinking, suggests two reasons. First, people develop routines — thought paths that get them efficiently through the day. Without such routines it would be impossible to get very much accomplished. Secondly, it is our own attitudes (thoughts or feelings that spring from our belief systems) that prevent us from being creative. Von Oech calls these "mental locks," defining them as "certain attitudes which lock our thinking into the status quo and keep us thinking 'more of the same.'" It is hard to be creative if our thinking is under the influence of any of these. He identifies the following 10 "mental locks" and then refutes them:

↦ teacher vs. therapist

1. **The Right Answer.** Our educational system often stresses this, and it becomes deeply ingrained in our thinking. Real life, though, is more complex and there may in fact be many "right" answers.

2. **That's Not Logical.** So called "lateral thinking" makes connections across diverse categories and not just within one, generating many novel concepts and ideas.

3. **Follow the Rules.** Rules often are arbitrary — they can be changed, broken or bettered. Rules help us become socialized but can keep us playing games that are very limiting.

4. **Be Practical.** Probing the possible, the impossible and the impractical for ideas is often fruitful. Why spend hours on a model airplane or a drawing? Why fly to the moon? This kind of thinking gets us nowhere. Don't limit the imagination when first approaching a problem — brainstorm.
5. **Avoid Ambiguity.** In real life, this is difficult. There is often more than one meaning or interpretation to an object, an event or a person's actions that forces a person to stretch his/her thinking and reach a deeper understanding of what's going on.
6. **To Err is Wrong.** Learning from mistakes can be as valuable, if not more so, than avoiding them.
7. **Play is Frivolous.** Play is necessary — it activates a different part of the brain, and expands thinking.
8. **That's Not My Area.** Limiting the scope of one's knowledge and experience can limit creativity. Crossing boundaries and transferring knowledge from one area to another can bring fresh insights to a field.
9. **Don't Be Foolish.** Giving oneself license to play the fool shakes up thinking and generates ideas and fresh perspectives.
10. **I'm Not Creative.** Too often a self-fulfilling prophecy.

Creative Expression and Our Clients

Many books on becoming more creative are filled with ideas for exercises and experiences that are fun and helpful. These are worth examining as a means of sparking creativity. Some of them may also be useful to our clients in the difficult task of breaking down barriers to creativity. Attitudes (such as the ones discussed above) plus feelings (e.g., fears of failure or of looking foolish) that support these attitudes can be very resistant to change. How can the therapist help foster creativity?

Helping clients express creativity involves recognizing and slowly chiseling away at these attitudes when they arise. When clients say they aren't creative, rather than contradicting this creative block, point out ways in which they have already successfully demonstrated their creativity. This may be in the formal sense (a poem, a painting) or informally (putting together an outfit, cooking, doodling).

Provide a balance between structured activities (where the outcome is more directed and manageable) and open-ended activities (in which the outcome rests more heavily on the individual).

Be respectful and compassionate but persistent in dealing with clients' fears regarding creative expression. Fears are real for those who experience them. Many clients have recently experienced a loss, creating fears of the unknown or unexpected. Explain to the client that the trick with fears is often to wait them out rather than running away from them. Stand firm and with time they will take on a more manageable form or perhaps even shrink away to nothing. Patience is important.

Everyone experiences creative impasses. A normally enthusiastic participant will suddenly become a stuck and bored individual. Sometimes people can't explain their feelings or don't understand how to move through this state. Try doing something different to change perspective. For example, if you are running a visual arts program, go on an outing and take sketch pads (the zoo is a great place to draw). For a music therapy program, bring in an assortment of junk and suggest that clients recycle it into musical instruments. As a last resort, walk or crawl backwards just to see things in a new way.

Be playful and have fun. Playfulness and creativity are intertwined. Believe that clients are creative and they will live up to this expectation.

Enhancing or Hindering Expression in Groups

In a group situation there are three elements that influence creative expression: the therapist, the environment and members of the group.

Although it is ideal when each of these elements helps enhance expression, it is often enough if weaknesses in one area are compensated for by strengths in the others. A skilled therapist may bring out the best in a group despite limited materials or inadequate space and can still teach clients how to be effective group members.

Qualities That Enhance Expression:

The **therapist** enhances expression by exhibiting the following qualities:

- **Authenticity.** Staying real — being able to react honestly to a situation without masking feelings.
- **Understanding.** A potent quality; a client who feels that s/he has been heard and accepted is likely to feel that s/he can express his/her own individuality and creativity.
- **Respect for privacy.** Being receptive to what clients are willing to disclose/not disclose.
- **Being comfortable with him/herself and the group.** Increases the chance that everyone else will relax and be comfortable as well.
- **A non-judgmental attitude and objectivity.** Both qualities encourage people to express their individual viewpoints.
- **Supportive guidance.** An attitude which fosters self-reliance and risk taking behaviors in the group.
- **Ability to create a feeling of partnership.** A feeling that "we are all in this together" creates a group bond which facilitates sharing, cooperation and a sense of participation in each other's growth and discovery.
- **Enthusiasm.** An infectious quality which often energizes group members.
- **Sincerity.** "Say what you mean, mean what you say;" this creates trust in the group.

- **Warmth and caring.** Nurturing clients may enable them to open up in ways that they would be reluctant to do in a less supportive environment.
- **Understanding psychological safety.** Knowing what creates a perception of safety and how to provide ground rules that support this perception.
- **Respect for each person's own pace.** Being aware that there will be different rates at which group members learn, share and become comfortable with others and new situations. Not forcing a pace.
- **Participation.** Being an active group member and/or modeling participation when necessary.
- **Playfulness.** This modeling by the therapist permits a spirit of playfulness in the group.
- **A neutral position.** The therapist does not become enmeshed in group dynamics but stays on the outside.

Environmental qualities that enhances expression:
- **A variety of good materials.** Provide the best materials possible (given the circumstances of budget and availability) and maintain all tools (scissors, glue, etc.) in good working order.
- **Provide choices.** Individual choice is what lies at the core of leisure. The more options offered, the more empowered the group will be.
- **Availability of inside/outside environment.** Most facilities have a "recreation or art room" — but using a patio, courtyard or even a park setting for a program can be exhilarating for clients. (Suzanne Mirviss: "One of my memorable experiences with clients was combining a beach picnic with art and music. We made sand candles, then a huge sand castle, sang and let our senses absorb the ocean world. There was room to expand because there were no walls to close us in.")
- **Colorful space.** If the group meets in an institutional setting there probably are restrictions on what can be changed in the

environment (e.g., painting walls). Have at least a board to display artwork and/or a locked glass display case.

- **Adequate lighting.** Enough lighting must be available, particularly for those with visual disabilities, to be able to work properly.
- **Appropriate music.** Tastes will differ, but select music that is appropriate to the setting, group and activity.
- **Few distractions.** Elicit staff help in eliminating as many outside distractions as possible. Radios, television and people traffic in and out of a room can all hinder creative expression.
- **Workspace.** Keep spaces clean and uncluttered. Allow room to spread out and work. Make sure everyone can establish an adequate personal space.
- **Space.** One that allows for closeness and distance, openness and privacy. Space in which to move and expand when it is called for, yet also space for retreat if someone needs it.

Members of the group help enhance expression through their:

- **Support.** Group members should be encouraged to be supportive, not negative. Negative feelings damage group cohesiveness.
- **Acceptance.** All members, including the therapist, need to feel accepted into the group in order for the group to function effectively.
- **Willingness to share ideas/feedback.** Members need to be active participants (most of the time) in order for the group to progress and be fruitful. There may be times when this is not psychologically possible, in which case a person's mental state should be respected.
- **Commitment to being there.** This should be established in the early stages of the group. When members do not show up, their absence affects the rest of the group.

- **Ability to work with the therapist and each other.** A member cannot function if there isn't the ability/desire to work within the established structure.
- **Willingness to engage in the creative process.** If a member doesn't really want to be in the group and/or isn't interested in the activities, it wastes everyone's time and energy.

Qualities that Hinder Expression:

Needless to say, it is important to try to minimize the number of these factors that are operating in the group.

A therapist may hinder expression in the following ways:
- **Criticism.** Find ways to make positive suggestions rather than criticize.
- **Too much or too little structure.** Too much structure and people feel trapped; too little and they flounder. Create enough structure to allow people room to explore with a purpose.
- **Too much or too little direction.** A balance must be struck so that clients don't end up feeling babied or, at the opposite extreme, feeling lost. Continually evaluate the level of the clients' needs for direction.
- **Inappropriate sharing of self.** Know professional boundaries and share only what is needed.
- **Distance.** Being psychologically disengaged or inaccessible to the group, standing apart from group activities.
- **Disrespect for clients' needs.** Not being client-focused in goals and interactions, but imposing goals and expectations.
- **Lack of encouragement.** Without encouragement, confidence may remain low in clients tackling new creative activities.
- **Lack of preparation.** The group's perception will be that they or the activity are not very important to the therapist, though this may far from true. A one-time problem will not be harmful, being chronically underprepared will.

- **Absence of feedback.** Without feedback on their individual projects and contributions to the group, members may feel their efforts are worthless and underappreciated.
- **Forcing exposure/interpretation.** This is associated with "disrespect for clients' needs." Forcing is not only psychologically painful but counterproductive to creative work.
- **Pushing the process.** Any new process must have time in which to evolve. Efforts to push it in a particular direction or speed it up will usually fail. The therapist who shows patience in letting the process develop will be rewarded with greater (and perhaps unexpected) results.
- **Insincerity.** Clients can usually identify staff who are not sincere. Often this is interpreted as a lack of respect for the client — a definite block to create expression.

Negative factor in the **Environment** may be

- **Formality.** An overly formal setting discourages clients from feeling that they can be playful, messy and/or relaxed.
- **Sterility.** An cold and empty space will be barren and unstimulating for clients trying to engage in creative work.
- **Lack of necessary time.** Planning is *critical*. Clients' stress levels rise when they feel rushed. Stress can reduce the ability to be creative. (In some cases, clients are habitually slow as this gets them attention from others. In this situation, it is best to deal with structuring time right from the beginning.)
- **Uncomfortable space.** A cramped, cluttered or dirty space can be physically and/or psychologically unpleasant for clients. Being too cold or too hot, feeling unsafe or uncomfortable all stop the "creative juices." Maslow (1968) clearly outlined the need for us to deal with human comforts before we can experience creativity.
- **Noise and/or distractions.** These make it difficult to concentrate. Creativity is best experienced in a state of "flow." Numerous distractions make it difficult to sustain this state.

Members of the group may hinder creative expression through:

- **Pre-conceived ideas.** Did the member come into the group with an inaccurate picture of the group's purpose and plan?
- **Negative feelings.** Negativity becomes a wall unless the therapist deals with the feelings.
- **Depression or fatigue.** Members in either of these states may cast a heavy shadow over the group. Know group members and check in regularly to see how they are doing. They may need time away from the group to sort out feelings.
- **Disrespect.** Damages self-esteem (collective or individual) and creates anxiety.
- **Lack of confidence.** Based on fears like "I'm not creative" this can hold back both individuals and groups.
- **Fear of exposure/interpretation.** These fears can make self-expression a nearly impossible task and must be dealt with by the therapist and the individual.

3

Roles of the Therapist

The therapist who uses the arts as therapeutic tools with groups embarks on a journey of discovery and wonder. Even with the most meticulous planning there is an element of mystery regarding what will emerge from the minds and spirits of the individuals in a group. It is the magic of the arts to touch the spirit and promote a level of communication that is different from everyday life. The therapist who is willing to design the opportunity for creative expression and recognize and use the information that emerges to a therapeutic end must be able to take on diverse roles, not the least of which is being a willing traveler in a realm that is ever provocative and mysterious. In order to gird him/herself for this journey, it is important that the therapist examine the variety of roles s/he must be comfortable assuming in this therapeutic process. His/her primary roles will be those of facilitator, teacher, artist and therapist.

The Role of Facilitator

To "facilitate" or "ease the way" requires giving up the therapist's traditional position as the only knowledgeable authority in the group.

It is important to create a group climate where members feel they can derive support from one another as well as the therapist. Since creative experience is often an enigma, it puts all group members on equal ground by its very nature, each trying to grasp its meaning. An effective facilitator will enable clients to be authorities on what is true for them, give and receive information and support each other's growth and discovery.

Being an effective facilitator means being able to:

Create **safety** within the group.

> In order for individuals to become truly functioning members of a group, it is important that they feel safe with each other. Specific ground rules need to be established at the start of the group dealing with how members will show respect to other group members, respond to each other in sharing their insights and feelings, participate and behave as vital members of the group. If the group environment is safe, then individuals are comfortable exploring and expressing what they discover in the art experience.

Be a **role model.**

> People often learn more from what is *done* than what is said. It is important not just to tell clients how to be effective members of the group, but to show them by example what that entails. Group members look to the therapist to *show* them, for example, how to give or receive feedback from others.

Participate.

As an effective role model, it is important to become an *active participant* in the group. Standing back and observing while members are engaged in an activity may be necessary in some circumstances but not helpful on a regular basis. As in the case of role modeling, participation is best facilitated by participating — doing the activities as a part of the group — rather than just talking about it.

Take risks.

To take risks means to invite change. In a group, a risk may be anything — from encouraging a client to say more about his/her work, to admitting to not knowing how to do something. Taking a risk and succeeding can encourage others to try taking more risks of their own. Paradoxically, clients who learn to see failure as non-fatal may be also feel encouraged to take risks. Even if the risk-taking is a failure, it may allow clients to see the therapist as human and accessible. By risking vulnerability the therapist opens him/herself to the possibility that s/he will be allowing other people to shine. This communicates a willingness to strengthen others' self-esteem — a powerful mechanism for accomplishing that task. (Suzanne Mirviss: "One of the most poignant moments I have ever had was taking the risk of admitting that I didn't know how to solve a problem with a group art project. That admission allowed a group member with some related experience to come forward and lead us through the dilemma.")

Be genuine.

If a person is not genuine, s/he is perceived as not trustworthy, which affects the climate of safety in the group. What the therapist says within the group should feel *real* to others. For example, if the therapist says to a client, "You're doing great!" when it is obvious that the individual isn't actually doing all that well, the individual may question the genuineness of the therapist and mistrust any subsequent feedback.

Be **friendly** and open to others.

Part of effective facilitating is to be a welcoming presence, friendly and genuinely happy to be there for clients. If a therapist is burned out or fears self-disclosure, for example, s/he will find it difficult to create a warm and supportive group environment. Being open to others, feeling honest compassion and caring what happens to people is the medicine of true healing.

Encourage **freedom within structure.**

One of the challenges of group work is to create a comfortable amount of structure for the group members (e.g., a plan of activities for each session) and still maintain a climate of freedom. Being flexible, paying attention to clients and being open to change of activities or direction allows clients to experience feelings of freedom. Many therapists have had the experience of coming to a group armed with what they felt were wonderful activities and have been met with blank stares that said, "I don't want to do this." The reasons may have little to do with the therapist (e.g., pain, adjustment of medications, lack of sleep). Effective facilitating means being willing to abandon a plan in favor of trying to discover what group members need.

Maintain proper **boundaries.**

A therapist needs to participate, take risks and have compassion, but s/he must also maintain proper personal boundaries. This means not crying over his/her own personal struggles or sharing his/her life history with clients. The clients, not the therapist, are there for help. Becoming socially involved with clients in a group can also jeopardize boundaries and confuse roles. Clients can't decipher where *friend* ends and *therapist* begins.

Be a **catalyst.**
A catalyst makes things happen. Many clients are over-whelmed by life changes or have a disability which impairs their ability to initiate action. Facilitating may at times mean being the "spark," providing the energy or ideas that will help clients initiate change in their lives.

The Role of Teacher

Being a teacher is an integral part of a being a therapist. The therapist who makes use of the creative arts will be actively in-volved in instructing, demonstrating, evaluating and looking for new ideas in order to motivate clients.

The **teacher** needs to know:

How people **learn.**
In order to be client-focused (gauging the growth of our clients as measure of our success) we need to understand that people learn in different ways. Some are visual learners who need to see information before them in order to learn it. Others are auditory (hearing) learners who learn and remember best through what they hear. Kinesthetic learners learn by doing. Most people have one or more areas of strength. A skilled teacher recognizes that everyone learns differently and tries to address more than one learning style when teaching an activity.

Presentation of activities and materials.
Presentation refers both to the style of the teacher and the tim-ing and methods of introducing activities. A quiet activity may need to follow a high-energy one. Activities which may impact clients emotionally may need to be introduced slowly and be preceded by warm-up activities.

There are many effective styles of presentation. Some teachers are exuberant and create that kind of energy in a group; some quietly command attention. Regardless of style, the following techniques apply:

- Say what needs to be said in several different ways and at different intervals in order to make sure clients understand what they need to know.
- Summarize what has been said.
- Practice using techniques and materials in advance of using them in the group — familiarity will save time and prevent mistakes.

Resources and techniques.
A "grab bag" of ideas and techniques will allow the therapist to be flexible and responsive to group needs. Keeping up to date on new developments in the field and creating an expanding repertoire of ideas and activities will increase the therapist's effectiveness as a teacher.

How to be a learner as well as a teacher.
The best teachers are those that love to learn. To inspire the love of learning and the desire to explore new ideas is a great gift to those in our care. The teacher who is a learner is also sensitive to what it feels like *not* to know, which is a vulnerability that every learner experiences. This knowledge can motivate you to find effective ways of helping clients grasp what you are teaching them.

The Role of Artist

Is it necessary to be a painter, musician or other accomplished artist to use the arts as therapeutic tools? Feeling that they are not creative is often a concern of therapists who are interested in the arts but aren't comfortable or don't feel capable of successfully leading arts-based therapeutic activities. While it certainly helps to have expertise in some aspect of the arts, it isn't mandatory in order to incorporate them into group work. What *is* needed is a clear idea of what the arts can accomplish for clients and the ability to see oneself as a facilitator of creative expression.

The **"artist"** needs to:

Believe that everyone has the need, right and ability to express creativity in their lives.

People are naturally creative. As children we are encouraged to use art materials, explore our ideas, feel free with creativity. At some point, many people receive the message that other activities are more important than creative activity and their energy is diverted away from the arts. Some people receive damaging messages like, "You'll never be an artist." or "You have to be really talented to succeed in the arts, work on practical skills." What results is a culture of people cut off from an important aspect of themselves — and missing that passionate engagement they felt in childhood. Expressing creativity is a necessity for all human beings and our job is to find and use these avenues in order to assist our clients in healing and in attaining fulfillment.

Understand the **role of creativity** in everyday life.

Creativity, self-expression and playfulness go hand-in-hand. Daily activities can be seen from the perspective of the creative choices that are being made, from putting together clothes to developing ways of making clients comfortable in a new activity. Broadening the definition of the forms of creative expression can lead to an increased awareness of creative choices for the client.

Know his/her **barriers to creativity.**

A therapist needs to be aware of the blocks and negative messages that s/he may have about creativity. These messages affect our attitudes, infiltrate our being and cause doubt and fear. Finding ways to break down these barriers will enable the "artist" to better express his/her own creativity and help clients to do the same.

Explore the arts.

There is a virtually limitless supply of ideas, materials and processes. If one technique doesn't inspire the therapist and/or the group, there are many others to experiment with. A few suggestions for sources: books, craft magazines, newspapers, courses and the Internet.

The Role of Therapist

As therapists, we seek to enable our clients to live fuller, more balanced and joyful lives. One means of reaching this goal is by promoting the experience of leisure. Since the leisure experience itself touches every aspect of life, it is even more potently present during creative activity. We find that utilizing the tools of creativity becomes a natural avenue for therapeutic healing. Regardless of their therapeutic orientation, therapists may incorporate processes that come from a variety of allied health therapies such as art, psychology, drama, dance, music, recreational and occupational therapy.

In using processes from allied professions we must be clear about our professional goals and boundaries. An art therapist, for example, has specialized training primarily focused on psychology, art development and art modalities. S/he is qualified to interpret art, diagnose and recommend treatment. Drama therapy, dance therapy or music therapy also require specialized training and experience. All therapists are not necessarily qualified or trained to perform these functions. We can, however, use processes of the art or music therapist as material for exploration in groups. How we use these processes and how we deal with the information that emerges is different and must lie within the boundary of our own profession. For example, rather than interpreting a client's artwork we would have the client *tell us* what it means. We may discover something important about a client during a group and may take it to a treatment team meeting for information and discussion even if we ourselves cannot establish an art therapy or drama therapy treatment plan. It is our responsibility to remember our professional boundaries and also to appreciate our roles as therapists.

A **therapist** needs to know:

The **purpose** of the group.

Has the group formed to learn an art skill, to celebrate their lives, for personal exploration or for a more therapeutic goal? The purpose sets the tone of the group: the manner and style of the therapist, the interactions among all members of the group and the way information is gathered and processed within the group.

The **goals** of the group.

What should be accomplished during the duration of the group and ultimately by each client? Once the goals of the group have been clearly defined, it is possible to choose and incorporate creative arts activities that will be appropriate (intellectually and emotionally). Success in the group is directly related to clear and realistic goals.

Observation skills.

Just as clients learn from observing our actions, we learn from observing their behavior in the group. Good observation skills enable the therapist to catch an important body posture, a facial expression, an emotional reaction or a subtle behavior. These unconscious reactions are often more revealing than what people say with words.

Psychological development.

In order to recognize and understand the issues that clients may be dealing with, it is important to be familiar with the psychosocial tasks that individuals must work through during different stages of their lives and the impact that failure to resolve these issues may have on an individual's development.

Group dynamics.

A therapist who works with groups needs to understands how they function. Significant aspects of group dynamics include:
- how individuals become a group
- the stages of group development
- styles of leadership and their effect on the group
- conflict resolution
- how to be effective with the varying chemistry of groups

How to be **intuitive.**

What am I feeling? What is the client really asking for? What would bring closure to this group? Being intuitive is often referred to as a sixth sense, as an ability to read between the lines. It is not so much taught, as developed.

The concept of **"least restrictive intervention."**

Ones that allows the client to work out the process of personal change with as much freedom and personal expression as s/he and the group are comfortable with.

How to *not* **analyze.**

Participants will find their own answers in the images and work they produce and sometimes in verbalizing their private explanations. It may be enough to allow the client his/her own private insights and revelations without further explanation.

Priority setting.

Just as facilitating means creating freedom within structure, being an effective therapist means finding a balance between prescriptive activities and choice. Some activities have more therapeutic value and carry more therapeutic weight than others. Schedules may need to be rearranged to fit the psychological needs of members, but if the purpose of the group is to work through problems, there may be activities which cannot be presented as optional.

Activity analysis.

Activities should be carefully chosen to meet the goals of the group. Being knowledgeable about activity analysis allows a therapist to judge the physical, cognitive, emotional and social demands of activities that s/he might consider introducing to a group. Activity analysis can help answer questions such as: Is this activity age-appropriate? What knowledge, skills and abilities are required to complete the task? What leadership style will I assume? As therapists we should always plan and choose our interventions responsibly. Everything we do has an impact on the people with whom we work.

Leisure theory.

Understanding the importance of leisure as it is integrated into a person's experience enables the therapist to look for ways to empower clients so they can find their own answers about shaping their time and to express these in a way that gives them integrity and self-esteem.

4

The Individual and the Therapy Group

Every individual who joins a therapy group is a unique composite of personal experience, psychological development, personality, biology, culture, age, gender and physical circumstance. One of the challenges of creating any group is to understand how all these components impact the individual and the expectations and roles that s/he may play out within the group setting. This will in turn affect the "chemistry" of the group and how it functions.

Another challenge is to understand the relationship of the individual to the therapist (the "helping relationship") and the dynamics of a group — how individuals may interact and how the group process typically evolves through time. As therapists, we expect to be able to manage all the emotion and complexity of the group. But this is a complex puzzle — one that takes time to put together. This chapter presents several "pieces" of the puzzle, progressing from individual to group issues. To put it another way, it builds a framework for understanding the behavior of groups and the individuals that are part of them.

There are many ways to structure information so that the therapist can grasp the complex dynamics of interaction. The therapist must understand normal growth and development models of awareness, patterns of interaction, the stages of psychological development within therapy groups, the helping relationship and aspects of separation after engagement. This chapter provides the therapist with information on each of these topics, focusing on the way they make running a group easier.

Individuals in the Group

The process of understanding clients and their needs is complex and ongoing. Understanding what someone needs involves gathering information, conferring with other staff, listening to the client and observing his/her behavior. Our understanding of the client is dynamic and evolves as we continue to interact with the individual.

"Assessment" is the term for gathering information about clients in order to design a program which addresses their needs and interests. The keys to assessment are to *research, listen, observe and analyze*.

General information which can be gathered about an individual client includes:

- **age and gender.**
- what is the **length of time** this individual been at the facility and the length of time available to work with this individual?
- **level of social functioning** — how well does this individual function in a group setting? If relevant, what provokes negative responses or behaviors in the client? Has the treatment team established a consistent approach in response to the client's negative responses or behaviors?
- **nature of any disabilities and abilities**.
- **health status** — is the individual often in pain, on medication, or affected by a physical or mental condition? Is the person's general condition stable and predictable or erratic and somewhat unregulated?

- **interests** — current and past.
- **support systems** — what types of support does the client have outside of the facility? What types does s/he have inside the facility? Where will this client be discharged to?

In addition, the therapist will often interview prospective members of a group before the first meeting, to assess each person's behavior, interests and motivation for being in the group. The meeting is kept brief and friendly. This is where the skills of listening (for verbal clues) and observing (non-verbal behavior) come into play.

Stages of Development

The line of life is like a flowing river. At the head of the river, water flows in small, shallow trickles. As the river flows to its end, the flow rate, depth and even the life existing in the water change. So is the progression of growing older and maturing. Individuals go through steps as they span the years. The charts on the following pages are meant to be an overview of typical growth and development milestones.

These milestones are only general guidelines. It is important to remember that a person's chronological age (how many years s/he has been alive) may be different than his/her biological age (how fast his/her body had aged) or his/her functional age (how his/her skills compare to the skills expected for different age groups).

Cultural norms and environment also impact an individual's development. Young girls in first world nations who have plenty (maybe too much) to eat tend to start puberty earlier than girls from third world countries who lack good nutrition. The life span of individuals within certain cultural and socioeconomic groups may be as much as thirty years longer because of lifestyle and health care options.

Probably the most important way in which developmental charts are to be used is to anticipate the individual's next step in the progression toward maturity and help prepare him/her for that step.

The following pages contain charts which are grouped by developmental age. Theorists like Piaget, Freud, Erikson, Kohlberg and Sullivan have all added to our understanding of the developmental process and their works have helped structure our developmental levels. The following charts include a short description of each of these theorist's ideas along with information about typical play behaviors, physiological events, common fears and medical preparation concerns for each developmental level.

Developmental levels do not end at adulthood. However, clear-cut levels are hard to scientifically support after the age of 20 years. After that point theorists provide "stages" of progression through such events as job maturity, retirement and death instead of developmental levels. It is for this reason that only Erikson's stages are provided.

Developmental Age: Birth to 12 Months

Psychosocial Stage of Development (Erikson)	*Stage One:* *Infancy*	Trust vs.	Ability to trust others and a sense of one's own trustworthiness; a sense of hope.
		Mistrust	Withdrawal and estrangement. Emotional dissatisfaction if needs have not been consistently met.
Moral Judgment (Kohlberg)	Kohlberg does not recognize a moral judgment awareness at this level.		
Radius of Significant Relationships (Sullivan)	*Maternal person* — may be either uni-polar or bipolar. Given the extent of child care used today, this distinction is slipping.		
Cognitive Stage (Piaget)	Piaget calls this stage the *sensorimotor stage* and extends the chronological age of this stage to two years.		
Psychosexual Stage (Freud)	*Oral-Sensory* — One of the major sources of pleasure from this age comes from exploring the world through oral activities such as vocalizing, sucking, chewing.		
Play Behaviors	Engages in playful activity alone and independently. Will engage in play with someone who is older but play behavior is centered around what interests him/her. Explores world visually by random movement. As ability to grasp and ability to put things in his/her mouth develops, explores the world this way also.		

Developmental Age: Birth to 12 Months

Basic Physiological Events	Develops basic control of body through space (hand to mouth, sitting up, pulls self to standing, crawling, roll from back to abdomen when lying down). Develops basic fine motor control (palmer grasp, radial-digital grasp, scissor grasp, 3-jaw chuck grasp and pincer grasp).
Common Fears	Loss of care/support from trusted adults, strangers, animals, loud noises, sudden movements and bright lights.
Medical Preparation Concerns[1]	Patients who are functionally under one year of age rely heavily on the support of a parent or familiar staff to survive unknown and scary situations. Explain the procedure to a parent or staff person who has a trusting relationship with the patient and is willing to stay with the patient through the procedure. Patients, lacking the general ability to control their environment, are soothed by the physical presence of a parent or staff person that they can trust. These patients are also extremely limited in their ability to adjust quickly to new environments. Provide the patient with familiar objects from his/her room along with the company of the parent or familiar staff person while the procedure is being performed.

---

[1] From burlingame and Skalko, **Idyll Arbor's Glossary for Therapists.** 1997. Idyll Arbor, Inc.

Developmental Age: 1 Year to 3 Years

Psychosocial Stage of Development (Erikson)	*Stage Two:* *Late infancy and early child- hood*	Auto- nomy vs. Shame and Doubt	Self-control without loss of self esteem; ability to co-operate and to express one-self. Compulsive self-restraint or compliance; defiance, willfulness. Shame. Doubt: feelings that nothing one does is any good.
Moral Judgment (Kohlberg)	*Pre-conventional* (pre-moral). External moral-ity, directed and imposed by authoritarian fig-ures. There are two levels associated with pre-conventional stage. The first one, punishment-and-obedience orientation (where actions are labeled as "good/bad" based on the conse-quences received), falls into this age group.		
Radius of Significant Relationships (Sullivan)	*Parental Persons* (tri-polar)		
Play Behavior	Plays alone and independently. Others may be playing nearby but their actions have little to moderate influence on the child's play.		
Psychosexual Stage (Freud)	*Anal Stage.* Individuals learn to withhold or expel fecal material at will. Future personality traits such as stinginess, stubbornness, expan-siveness, over-generosity and orderliness or messiness are developed and fine-tuned.		
Basic Physiological Events	Turns pages in books, can build a tower of blocks up to 9 blocks tall, walks up and down stairs, stands on one foot for a few seconds, in artwork is able to copy circles and crosses.		

Developmental Age: 1 Year to 3 Years

Common Fears	Separation from parent/primary care takers, injury, certain persons or locations (e.g., doctor, dentist office), loud or sudden noises, dark places, large machines.
Medical Preparation Concerns[2]	Patients rely heavily on the gross and fine motor ability that they have. Restricted movement may increase the patient's level of stress. Simple procedures like a blood pressure check may produce anxiety. For painless procedures, showing the equipment, performing the procedure on an anatomically correct doll or "teaching" the patient how to imitate the procedure on the doll may reduce fear. Play may need to be done a few times prior to the actual appointment. This group does not have an understanding of what is inside the body. Avoid lengthy discussions about what is going to be "fixed" or "examined." Concentrate on how the treatment/procedure will feel. Intense emotional upset and physical resistance is developmentally normal. A procedure should be done as quickly and gently as possible with a trusted staff person or parent physically close. After a painful procedure, numerous opportunities to "work out" fear and misunderstanding is appropriate. Frequently this group equates pain directly with punishment. If the patient is verbal and talks about the doll being "bad" or needing a time out prior to having the procedure, the staff can direct the patient's play to reflect a truer picture of what happened.

[2] From burlingame and Skalko, **Idyll Arbor's Glossary for Therapists.** 1997. Idyll Arbor, Inc.

Developmental Age: 3 to 6 Years

Psychosocial Stage of Development (Erikson)	*Stage Three:* *Early Childhood*	Initiative vs. Guilt	The courage to try to achieve desired goals tempered by a sense of conscience. Self-denial and self-restriction.
Moral Judgment (Kohlberg)	*Pre-conventional* (pre-moral). Morality is external, being directed and imposed by authoritarian figures. There are two levels associated with pre-conventional stage. The second one, the instrumental-relativist orientation (where behaviors are considered to be "right" if it brings pleasure), falls into this age group.		
Radius of Significant Relationships (Sullivan)	*Basic Family*		
Play Behavior	Child plays with toys; engages in activities similar to the others nearby, but plays next to, instead of with, others. Engages in make-believe and dramatic play.		
Psychosexual Stage (Freud)	*Phallic Stage.* Freud noted that it is during this developmental period that children begin to recognized that there are differences between the sexes. They also discover that their genitals are interesting and sensitive. He speculated that penis envy and castration anxiety were important concerns for children in this age group. Freud associated such personality traits as shyness/brashness, blind courage/timidity and stylishness/plainness as developing during this stage.		

Developmental Age: 3 to 6 Years

Basic Physiological Events	Skips and hops on one foot, throws and catches balls well, walks backward, ties shoelaces, uses seven to nine parts when drawing a stickman, constantly active.
Common Fears	Monsters, ghosts or other supernatural beings, injury, death, "bad" people, the dark.
Medical Preparation Concerns[3] (Material in this section is based on the developmental needs of patients between the ages of three years and seven years of age. Around the age of seven years children are more able to understand medical and health issues.)	(Ages 3 to 7 years.) Patients tend to think egocentrically and explain unknowns through magical thinking. Without adequate preparation, their minds can become quite active with imagination, making the procedure more exaggerated, bizarre and frightening than it actually is. Explain the procedure to them using dolls, puppets and other visual aids. Allow them to take the part of the practitioner prior to the procedure until they feel more relaxed. This reduces the need for both physical and chemical restraints. Children of this age tend to have concerns about mutilation, especially fears of castration. While some adults who function at this developmental age don't exhibit this behavior, many patients will still experience this fear. Be very explicit about the part of the body that the procedure will be done on. Frequently patients want to act like "grown men and women." To them this means that they are not allowed to express their fears, cry or even to scream. With the use of the puppets or dolls, staff can help the patient learn appropriate ways in which to express feelings.

---

[3] From burlingame and Skalko, **Idyll Arbor's Glossary for Therapists.** 1997. Idyll Arbor, Inc.

Developmental Age: 6 to 12 Years

Psychosocial Stage of Development (Erikson)	*Stage Four:*	Industry	Realization of competence, perseverance.
		vs.	
	Middle Child-hood	Inferiority	Feeling that one will never be "any good," withdrawal from school and peers.
Moral Judgment (Kohlberg)	*Conventional Stage* where conformity, loyalty and maintenance of social order is paramount. This stage, closely corresponds to the child's operational level of cognitive function. The two levels of this stage (stages 3 and 4, building upon earlier stages) are 3. the interpersonal concordance (one earns approval by following "norms" and being a good girl/good boy) and 4. the "law and order" orientation where following the rules set out by authority equals "correct" behavior.		
Radius of Significant Relationships (Sullivan)	*Neighborhood and School.*		
Play Behaviors	Plays with others in an organized manner for a purpose (e.g., sports teams, to make something). Feelings of belonging to the group. The youth plays a role (leader/follower) and the others support that role to some degree.		
Psychosexual Stage (Freud)	*Latency Period.* Freud identified this time of maturation to be one of polishing previously acquired personality traits and using one's energy to acquire knowledge.		

Developmental Age: 6 to 12 Years

Basic Physiological Events	Can follow three step commands, repeats performances to improve skill, prefers to play with members of own sex, dresses self completely, generally likes competition, pubescent changes may begin to develop.
Common Fears	Storms, the dark, staying alone, failure in school and tests, supernatural beings (esp. seen on TV or in movies), death.
Medical Preparation Concerns[4] (Material in this section is based on the developmental needs of patients between the ages of seven years and thirteen years of age. Around the age of thirteen years adolescents are confused with the physiological changes and also want to have a say in what happens.)	Patients who are able to function in this developmental category are at least somewhat aware of different illnesses and how people cannot live without certain body organs. When preparing this group for invasive procedures, explain the procedure in a non-hurried manner first. Some of the patients will ask many, many questions to gain a sense of control. Please be patient. Understanding what is going to happen will reduce the need for restraints. Use scientific terminology for body parts and medical procedures. Unlike patients functioning below seven years or above 13 years, this group of patients may be embarrassed by having other people know that dolls were used to explain the procedure. If they don't want to use dolls or similar training props, explain the procedure with pictures.

---

[4] From burlingame and Skalko, **Idyll Arbor's Glossary for Therapists.** 1997. Idyll Arbor, Inc.

Developmental Age: 12 to 19 Years

Psychosocial Stage of Development (Erikson)	*Stage Five: Adolescence & Post Adolescence. "Identity Crisis."*	Identity vs. Role Diffusion	Sexual maturation/individuation. Coherent sense of self; plans to actualize one's abilities. Feelings of confusion, indecisiveness, antisocial behavior.
Moral Judgment (Kohlberg)	*Postconventional.* Social-Contract, legalistic orientation. Moral judgment tends to reflect generally accepted social standards and follow community laws. Individuals tend to believe that they can influence change of standards if changes need to be made to increase fairness and rights to the community in general.		
Radius of Significant Relationships (Sullivan)	*Outgroups.* Relationships during this time period tend to be an outgrowth of previously developed close friendships, first with individuals of the same sex, then branching out to members of the opposite sex.		
Play Behaviors	Generally both sexes engage in activities which involve their peers; females tend to spend more time talking about "things" than the males. Sports, hobbies and entertainment (computer games, videos and music) tend to make up much of the adolescents "play behavior."		
Psychosexual Stage (Freud)	*Genital Stage.* This stage begins at the onset of puberty and the production of sexual hormones. While interactions tend to move toward developing a significant relationship, a major source of pleasure comes from sexual pleasures and tensions.		

Developmental Age: 12 to 19 Years

Basic Physiological Events	Top age group for participation in sports, developmentally a need for independence and freedom from authority, likely to take risks, very strong need for approval from peers, girls generally two years ahead of boys develop- mentally.
Common Fears	Social isolation, physical changes in body and own sexuality, divorce of parents, gossip, speaking in public, making mistakes in public.
Medical Preparation Concerns[5]	Use visual aids to provide visualization of the procedures. Include a description of the expected external appearance after the procedure if the patient's normal appearance will change (e.g., cast, stitches). Patients functioning at this developmental level prefer not to have any familiar staff or a parent with them as the procedures are being explained. Respect their wish for privacy. Additional feelings of control, which should reduce the need for restraints, can be gained by having the patients make their own appointments.

---

[5] From burlingame and Skalko, **Idyll Arbor's Glossary for Therapists.** 1997. Idyll Arbor, Inc.

Developmental Age: 18 to 25 Years

Psychosocial Stage of Development (Erikson)	*Stage Six:* *Early Adult-hood*	Intimacy vs.	Capacity for love as mutual devotion; commitment to work and relation-ships without loss of self.
		Isolation	Impersonal rela-tionships, preju-dice.

Developmental Age: 25 to 65 Years

Psychosocial Stage of Development (Erikson)	*Stage Seven:* *Adulthood. 40* *— mid-life* *crisis;* *42 - 65 middle* *age.*	Genera-tivity vs.	Creativity, produc-tivity, concern for others, next gen-eration.
		Stagnation	Self-indulgence, impoverishment of self.

Developmental Age: 65 Years Plus

Psychosocial Stage of Development (Erikson)	*Stage Eight: Old Age.* Possible loss of social and economic status, diminishing physical stamina, institutionalization, disengagement from commercial and professional activities; relative, family and friends may become more important.	Ego Integrity vs. Despair	Acceptance of the worth and uniqueness of one's life. Emotional integration. That enables one to honor the past while preparing to relinquish leadership to younger people. Sense of loss, contempt for others. Life has been too short to achieve one's desires and that it is too late to begin again.

Development of Artistic Skills

A knowledge of developmental levels in art is useful for a number of reasons. If the target group includes children, the therapist can choose activities and materials more appropriately and will have more realistic expectations about what the children in a particular age group can successfully accomplish. (Though even within an age-appropriate activity there will be variation in children's abilities. Some first-graders will struggle with tracing and cutting through an entire art session while others glide easily through these tasks and move on to the next phase of an activity.) Understanding stages of art development also aids the therapist in guiding the child or adult with emotional or developmental challenges. Art therapists are often able to pinpoint delays or interruptions in development by examining artwork.

Listed below is an overview of artistic tasks which are generally accomplished from ages one to seven. By age seven, most individuals have acquired basic art skills: experience in the use of a variety of media, drawing with lines, shapes and textures, cutting, tracing and pasting. During the "realistic stage," or beginning at ages seven to ten, children become more interested in representational art. By late childhood or early adolescence, children in our culture begin to master linear perspective or creating the illusion of three dimensional depth on a two dimensional surface (Winner, 1986). But it is the drawing of childhood which is the heart and soul of many people's experience with art.

Whole Arm Drawing   Age 1

At this age a child is engrossed in learning to walk and acquiring gross motor skills. Drawing, a fine motor skill, is performed by the one year old with little motor control, by making large motions with the whole arm.

Scribbles and Scribbling   Ages 2-3

This is a stage of pure exploration of the materials, colors and the movements of hand and wrist. Scribbles are the building blocks of children's art and lead to formation of more recognizable shapes. In the art of drawing there is a form of preliminary sketching called "gesture drawing" that might be thought of as controlled scribbling. The child has about 20 basic scribbles in his/her repertoire, and by adding color variations, a lot of exploring can be undertaken through scribbling. Scribbling is spontaneous, since a child at this age doesn't start out with a plan in mind. The child takes pleasure and interest in the pattern his/her markings make against a background.

Secrets of Shape   Ages 2-4

Discovering the hidden shapes within the scribbles: circles, ovals, squares, rectangles, triangles, odd shapes and crosses.

Art in Outline   Ages 3-4

The child grasps the crayon and with a single line, draws a form that s/he likes in scribbles. S/he now has the ability to outline a shape. For the child a shape is pleasing, so a child's response may include that fact that the drawing has, for example, nice lines or pretty circles. A child may scribble and proudly say, "This is a tractor, here are the wheels, here is the man." The adult's job is to listen, be enthusiastic and not impose direction on the child. It is a time when a child is his/her own art teacher/explorer.

The Child and Design   Ages 3-5

Almost from the moment they are able to draw shapes in outline form, children begin to combine the forms into designs. For example, a circle may be placed inside a square or vice versa. When a child uses more than two shapes, the combinations become almost unlimited. At this stage children are developing a real style of their own — with favorite colors and shapes, ways to begin artwork or fill the page. Three is a very confident age.

Mandalas, Suns and Radials   Ages 3-5

Radials can be common asterisks, plants with waving fronds, Fourth of July explosions, a sun, a mandala wheel or a smiling face. This stage is an important departure from which the child may proceed to draw human figures.

People, People, People   Ages 4-5

Often from drawings of the sun comes the human face. Children also begin to create their first image of a human — the universal "tadpole" — consisting of a circle and two lines for legs (Winner, 1986). At first the head is huge in relationship to the stick legs. At this stage the child is not trying to draw a human likeness but only to place things in a way that looks right and is personally pleasing to him/her.

Almost Pictures   Ages 4-6

Once children begin to draw people, their designs start taking shapes that adults recognize, for example a boat or flower. Drawings of the human figure are followed, after a while, by pictures of animals which stand up on two legs instead of crouching down on all fours.

There is great charm and fluidity in childhood drawings. Encouragement to create clouds with faces or animals standing on two legs is reserved for the pre-school child. Often artists wishing to bring back the imagery of childhood have to "...work hard to do consciously and deliberately what they once did effortlessly and because they had no choice." (Winner, 1986, p. 35) "I used to draw like Raphael," Picasso is quoted as saying, "but it has taken me a whole lifetime to learn to draw like children."

Around age five, as children develop intellectually, they become more interested in drawing representationally. There is a desire to picture something from their own lives, from stories read to them or from their fantasy world. This focus of drawing will naturally begin to evolve, without adult interpretation.

Pictures   Ages 5-7

Usually until the age of five or six a child's pictures do not begin to tell their own story. Now we can begin to see the house with flowers, a rainbow and a smiling sun — a picture of life as they see it.

While ability to complete fine motor tasks vary within an age group, generally children between five and seven have increased dexterity. They can draw within an outline and vary the pressure of their marks from lighter to heavier for different effects. They can use almost any art medium now.

This five to seven year old stage is one of the critical periods in a child's art development. The child who feels free to use the colors and basic shapes which please him/her will continue to grow artistically when s/he moves into more pictorial work. This is when adults begin to give children more "formulas" for making their art more representational. Often children lose interest in art at the age of seven because they feel the disapproval or lack of encouragement from adults who may try to press them into creating "neat and acceptable" art. Sometimes people abandon art in childhood only to rediscover it later in life in a new form.

There is, of course, much more to art than drawing. There is color, light, emotion, media — a myriad of techniques and combinations to explore in order to communicate an idea or feeling. This section on the development of artistic skills covers only a small set of developmental milestones associated with art.

Johari Windows: A Self-Awareness Model

Johari windows are a way of representing how aware a person is of him/herself and how aware other people are of him/her. To use the model you ask yourself two questions:
- How well does this person know him/herself?
- How well do other people in the group know this person?

From those answers you can create a Johari window. Draw a box to represent the person. Draw a line from the top to the bottom of the box to represent the relative amounts the person knows about him/herself versus the amount that s/he does not know. Then draw a horizontal line from the left to the right to represent how much other members of the group know about the person versus how much they do not know. Obviously the lines will move during treatment as the group learns more about the person and the person learns more about him/herself.

There are four quadrants in the box as shown in the diagram below. Q1 (open) is information that is known to both the person and the group. It is called open because it is information that everybody knows. Q2 (blind) is information that the group has discovered that the person is still not aware of. A person's addiction which s/he is in denial about is one possible kind of knowledge that goes in this quadrant. Q3 (hidden) is information that the person knows about but has not shared. Q4 (unknown) is information that no one is aware of yet. Repressed memory would be in this quadrant.

	Known to self	**Not known to self**
Known to others	Q1 Open	Q2 Blind
Not known to others	Q3 Hidden	Q4 Unknown

Johari windows are useful for thinking about the dynamics of a group because they provide a graphic representation of the amount of sharing that a person has done and the amount of understanding a person has into his/her problems. In most therapeutic groups it is necessary to understand who is willing to share and who is not. It is also important to consider whether the person has the self-awareness to be able to share. The course of treatment is very different depending on the situation.

In the group shown below you can see several patterns. Laura is the most open because she knows a lot about herself and has shared it with the group. Maria and Sam both have very little open information, but the reasons are quite different. Maria knows a great deal about herself but is not willing to share it. Sam doesn't understand himself well, so even if he were willing to share information, he would not have very much to share. In the course of treatment the therapist would probably want to work with Sam on self-awareness and with Maria on being willing to share — two very different directions in therapy even though the problem of not sharing with the group is the same.

Group Awareness Configuration

Debbie

1	2
3	4

Laura

1	2
3	4

Sam

1	2
3	4

Van

1	2
3	4

Maria

1	2
3	4

Interaction Patterns

Any activity can be classified as belonging to an "interaction pattern." What follows is a progression of interaction levels. A psychologically healthy person can interact on all these levels. First start a person or group at the interaction level they are comfortable with. Program activities to generate success at the next higher level. This process allows for sequencing of activities for building social and interactional skills.

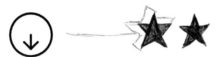

Internal

Action taking place within the mind or action involving the mind and a part of the body.

- requires no interactions or contact with another person or external object
- normal behavior unless taken to extreme

Examples: Twiddling thumbs, scratching your nose, fantasies, day dreaming, meditation, yoga

Problematic Behavior: Characterized by internal activities taken to the extreme. Potential groups which may have problems include children who are autistic, adults with psychiatric diagnoses such as severe depression, psychosis or schizophrenia, individuals with moderate to severe mental retardation exhibiting self-injurious behaviors.

Object-Oriented

Action directed by a person towards an object.

- requires interaction or contact with an object but not another person.

- requires awareness of and interest in inanimate objects.

Examples: Jigsaw puzzles, solitaire, pogo stick jumping, knitting, weight lifting, punching bag, watching TV, reading, arts, crafts, interacting with animals, guided imagery, tape visualizations, walking, computer games, gardening, individual creative arts activities.

Problematic Behavior: Characterized by an interaction based on compulsive behavior instead of interest or an extreme amount of time spent in object-oriented activities to the detriment of other levels. Potential groups include individuals with compulsive disorders, mental retardation (especially moderate to severe levels), dementias, autism or individuals with pathological patterns of computer or television use.

Aggregate

Action directed by a person toward an object while in the company of other persons who are also directing actions towards objects; physical proximity may allow for interaction, spontaneity, parallel play.

- action is not directed toward each other; no interaction between participants is required or necessary; may respond to leader.
- typical of large group leisure activities including spectator sports, aerobics classes, pedagogical learning activities and performance activities.

Examples: Bingo, roulette, watching movie, watching a play, crafts, mind assisted therapy, gardening, walking, watching a baseball game, many classroom situations, step-aerobics.

Problematic Behavior: Characterized by an individual who, for the most part, ignores other participants and only pays attention to "the leader" to the detriment of other participants. May be seen with some sensory input disorders including hearing impairment, some types of attention deficit disorders. May also be seen in individuals who feel acutely uncomfortable in social situations.

Inter-Individual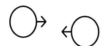

Action directed by one person toward another. It may or may not be competitive. The first didactic relationship. Ability to interact continuously with another; may be cooperative. If the focus is competition, may simulate inter-personal encounters in which individuals need to stand up for themselves against other persons.

- when the pattern is competitive, has the quality of assisting people to deal with stress, pressure and concepts of winning and losing; therapist must focus on this part and plan accordingly.
- continuous losing is not beneficial.
- characteristic of these activities is playing by the rules and regulating one's behavior according to the rules; to participate successfully, players agree to behave in certain ways.

Examples: Chess, checkers, tennis, ping pong, wrestling, mirroring, cooperative drawing, leader/follower, one-to-one conversations.

Problematic Behavior: At times there is a fine line between individuals who are pathologically inadequate in this skill and individuals who are making "normal" errors in interaction. While inter-individual interactions occur for most of us on a daily basis, this is an extremely complex process of sending messages and receiving feedback both verbally and with body language. An individual's expectations as s/he enters an interaction, his/her level of commitment to pay attention to what is said and his/her ability/desire to adhere to social norms all play a part. Some individuals may just be "etregenous." In this case the "sender" of the message has his/her train of thought momentarily interrupted because of the response s/he receives. The sender can tell that the receiver is on about the "same page" but can't figure out how the receiver logically came up with the response. More extreme are individuals with thought process disorders such as aphasia, hallucinations or who have vocal tics.

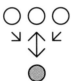

Unilateral

Action among three or more persons, one of whom is the antagonist or "it." Beginning of role differentiation.

- interaction consists of simultaneous didactic relationships vying for leader's attention.

Examples: Tag, dodge ball, black jack, Simon says, red light/green light, group mirroring with a leader, psychodrama, appreciation line-up, children vying for a parent's attention.

Problematic Behavior: Characterized by exceptional attempts to obtain the antagonist's attention — frequently seen in sociopathic disorders; potentially in individuals with head injury or perseveration disorders.

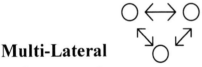

Multi-Lateral

Action among three or more persons, with no one person as an antagonist. Give and take from a lot of people at the same time. Having to react and/or initiate. Requires each person to initiate with the others.

- activities of this kind allow for a diffusion of effort.
- must deal with interaction from a number of people simultaneously as in life situations.
- responsibility for control is on each individual: decision making, strategy, action not shared by team members; requires a feeling of self-sufficiency.

Examples: Scrabble, Monopoly, poker game, group machine, encounter groups, theater games, casual socializing (e.g., "going out for coffee").

Problematic Behavior: Characterized by the individual who cannot tolerate sustained competitive/cooperative action with just one person.

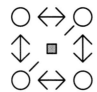

Intra-Group

Action of a cooperative nature by two or more persons intent upon reaching a mutual goal.

- action requires positive verbal or non-verbal interaction.
- helps to build social skills; may require compromise and cooperation.

Examples: Choir singing, orchestra playing, group dancing (e.g., the Hora), service projects, building a human pyramid, group puzzle, mural creation.

Problematic Behavior: Characterized by individuals who *must* have group cooperation or input when individualized responses are more appropriate or by individuals who have difficulty interacting with more than one person at a time. Individuals with sociopathic personalities have a hard time working in an Intra-Group setting.

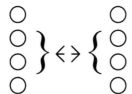

Inter-Group

Actions of a competitive or noncompetitive nature between two or more intra-groups.

- most difficult to perform since participants must cooperate with other team members and may compete with other team(s).

- action requires cooperation with some — competition with others.
- most complicated, many not ready for this level of interaction.
- may produce peer pressure which can be beneficial.

Examples: Scrounge, "laugh it up," basketball, football, charades, team sports, many vocational settings.

Problematic Behavior: As with the inter-individual level, there is a fine line between individuals who are making "normal" errors in the cooperation/competition required at this level. Group norms or expectations, rather than exact universal measurements, determine acceptable levels of performance at this level. Individuals who exhibit significant undesired behaviors which impede the performance of the others are demonstrating problematic behaviors.

Therapy Groups:
Stages of Psychological Development

There are predictable stages or phases of working with individuals, families or groups. Each group will have an initial, middle and ending phase. It is important to have some idea about what might be likely to happen and the sequence in which it normally unfolds. As the length of time allowed for treatment shortens due to managed care, it is harder for the therapist to move clients successfully through each phase. For this reason it is vital for the therapist to understand this sequence and know how to facilitate a smooth, continuous progression for each client. There is no longer enough time in treatment for the therapist to work without purpose. Several of the issues that are listed here are dealt with in more depth in the next section, *The Helping Relationship*.

Initial Phase: Development of Trust in Structure and Therapist

- Establishment of a "therapeutic alliance."

- Clarification of roles.
- Clarification of the nature of work to be done together.
- Conditions and structure for the group to work together.
- Group agreements: agreements made by the group and/or requests made by the group and/or by the therapist.
- Setting of firm, clear, consistent behavioral limits.
- Therapist gaining increased understanding of client(s).
- Enhancement of comfort level: the supportive phase.
- What to call the group (optional).

Middle Phase: Evoking Expression and "Working Through"

- Development of trust in other group members: The progression of trust may be rapid for some, slow for others — respect each person's pace.
- Periods of resistance: An inability or unwillingness to reflect or to engage, limited self-disclosure, superficial disclosure and/or regression. Resistance may be seen as a natural defense mechanism, a way to protect the self.
- Transference/Counter-transference issues.
- Process of risking, exploration and confrontation of ideas and affects (attitudes). Looking many times at the same issues. This is the period of facing, understanding, and, perhaps, accepting a problem.
- Cyclicity: An "open" session will often be followed by a "closed" session. There should be a sustained, empathic reminder by the therapist that people experience a great depth of anxiety regarding change. It is as if the psyche needs to balance disclosure with closure. The therapist wants to help sustain the tension of this "working through" phase.
- Change takes *time*; it is best if the therapeutic contact can continue long enough for genuine "working through" to occur. Defenses may re-emerge. Clients may experience inertia.

Ending Phase: Termination Process

- Penultimate Stage: Consolidation
    - Development and integration of a new image or definition of the self. Practicing new ways of behaving, mourning of the old ways and old fantasies.
    - A separation is in process (of therapist and group) which may be emotionally charged. There is possible re-experiencing of past separations.
- Termination
    - Why is it happening — is this a natural process or does it have other causes (insurance cuts, a program discontinued, parents withdraw a child)?
    - The therapist may review or summarize the therapy process and/or make referrals for continuation with another group/therapist.
    - Recognizing completion of the process or that this is as far as the client(s) can go, or may choose to go for now.
    - Client re-defining his/her role separate from support offered by the therapist.

The Helping Relationship

A professional "helping relationship" is a very unique association of two people, with its own set of rules and expectations. Unlike a friendship, it concentrates on meeting the needs of only one person — the client. The therapist is expected to have the knowledge and skills to assist the client in meeting a problem or a need and to accomplish what s/he could not do alone. The focus is on *assisting*; the therapist doesn't problem solve *for* the client but rather helps the client to grow psychologically and cognitively and become more self-sufficient.

How does a helping relationship develop and how is it maintained? Both the therapist and the client need to be willing to engage in certain behaviors that will ensure that a helping relationship will be productive. There are two basic phases to the helping relationship: the first phase is the building of the relationship, the second is the facilitation of a positive change in the client. Each phase tends to progress through about four different stages. These eight stages of a helping relationship are described below. Though much of the advice in this section is addressed to the therapist, there are areas (particularly Stage III) that address concerns of the client as well, and which might be shared with the client(s), if appropriate, at the start of the group.

Initial Phase: Building Relationships

1. Entry: Opening the Relationship (Cornerstones of the Therapeutic Alliance)

- Open the meeting.
- Help to create an environment where individuals may, as clearly as they are able, feel free to state needs, requests for help and invitations to work together.
- Assess: How do the individuals regard "being helped?" Is asking for "help" seen as a weakness?
- Remember that there is a natural reluctance in people to confront their feelings.
- Note the distance between chairs.
- Remember that psychological discomfort must be great for some before they seek assistance.
- Make use of indirect questions and statements:
  - "Please tell me what is on your mind."
  - "What do you wish to discuss with me?"
  - "I'm interested in knowing how you are, please fill me in."
- Remember, some situations seem too overwhelming or too unique for clients to share easily.
- Be aware of cultural implications regarding sharing of vulnerabilities.

- Some clients will be better able to disclose information if there is some object (e.g., a nerf ball or Rubik's cube) nearby which is acceptable for them to pick up and "play" with. This seems to help release some nervous energy.

2. Clarification: Reasons for Seeking Help (Statement of Problem or Concern)

- Be mindful of all questions; the individual may feel interrogated. Asking for elaboration on a situation and "how" questions may be helpful.
- Evaluate the degree of desire and motivation for change in the client(s).
- Is there an awareness of the potentials and limitations of a helping relationship?
- Many clients will not reveal the "true" problem or need until they present some superficial problems to see how the therapist reacts. Trust may need to be established through this process before the client is willing to reveal his/her primary concern.

3. Structure: Formulating the Contract and the Structure

- What are the conditions under which we will work?
- The goal for this (initial) stage is to decide whether to proceed.
- The following questions need to be answered by both parties:

Therapist Questions:
- Do I want to work with this person/group (comfort, compatibility)?
- Can I meet his/her expectations (given my skills, knowledge)?
- What am I expecting (time, place, effort, commitment, responsibility)?

- What kind of structure do we need to proceed (informal understanding, counseling contract or leave the issue open)?
- Am I able to work with this person/group (skills, knowledge, experience)? Do my intellect, intuition and heart agree?

Client Questions:
- Am I willing to commit myself to a relationship agreement, and if so, will we work it out together?
- Will this relationship get me more involved than I want to be?
- Will this person be helpful on my terms?
- What are his/her terms?
- Is this person able to understand who I am, my culture, my closely held beliefs? Will we be able to work on my agenda — not the therapist's agenda?
- If I agree to a "contract" to do specific things, can I get out of it if I want to?
- Is this a person I can trust?

4. Relationship: Building the Helping Relationship

- A gradual but steady increase in the depth of the relationship.
- A commitment has been made by the client and the therapist to work for change together. A level of trust has been reached.
- Stages 1-4 involve the therapist's growing to understand how the client(s) sees the world, through listening, clarifying and structuring information coming from the client.

Middle Phase: Facilitating Positive Action

5. Exploration: Exploring Problems, Formulating Goals, Planning Strategies, Gathering Facts, Expressing Deeper Feelings, Learning New Skills

- Therapist may become more active and assertive.
- There is a strong tendency on the part of the client to turn inward when describing feeling and delineating problems.
- Sometimes the client "feels so good" and experiences a "flight into health."
- Issues of transference (attitudes towards the therapist which have been transferred from earlier attitudes towards important figures in the client's life) and counter-transference (therapist towards client) emerge. Freud said that transference can be a therapist's most effective tool. It can help the client recapture the past by re-experiencing and enacting feelings.
- The specific process goals for the therapist at this stage are as follows:
  - Maintain and enhance the relationship (trust, ease, safety).
  - Deal with feelings that interfere with progress towards goals.
  - Encourage the exploration of feelings so that the client's self-awareness is expanded.
  - Gather necessary facts that will contribute to the solution of the problem.
  - Decide to continue or terminate the relationship.
  - Teach skills required to reach goals (demonstrating, modeling, coaching).
  - Initiate homework activities that move towards goals.

6. Consolidation: Exploring Alternatives, Working through Feelings, Practicing New Skills, Breaking Old Patterns

- A broadening of the client's perspective and world view takes place.
- A realization on the part of the client that past ways of thinking and acting did not work. Some trepidation mixed with excitement about trying new things causes the client to struggle anew.
- This is the point at which the client must decide to act or not, to operationalize the insights gained into his/her behavior.
- This can be a "Catch 22:" if clients change, they won't need the therapist or feel that the therapist will reject them because they don't need him/her any more.

7. Planning for the Future: Planning Strategies to Resolve Conflicts, Reducing Painful Feelings, Generalizing New Skills or Behaviors to Continue Self-Directed Activities

- Plans for termination/discharge and continuing alone are formulated.
- Goals for this stage are to crystallize discussions of earlier stages into a plan of action and to decide that growth has proceed to the point where termination of the relationship is indicated.
- Best results and decreased readmission/relapse tend to occur if the client has "practiced" (at least once) alternative modes of thought or behavior in the community, with the therapist's support. (In cases where the helping relationship was established when client was an inpatient).
- Bringing up new topics is discouraged.

Ending Phase: Termination Process

8. Termination

- Summarizing the process.
- Evaluating the outcomes.
- There are many methods of termination. The therapist:
  - may spread out sessions over a period of time to de-escalate the involvement (decrease frequency).
  - may want to leave the door open for follow-up.
  - may refer the client(s) to another therapist/agency/networking.

Activities/Rituals for Dealing with Separation

A variety of activities can be used to mark the ending of the therapy group. In addition to the following ones, many of the closure activities in other sections of the book (*Drama* or *Poetry and Writing*) would also be appropriate to use at this point in the group.

Gift
Each participant receives gifts from the group. Participants are sitting in circle. The one who speaks uses the format "I give you the gift of — ." The gift may be a wish for something material or something abstract; a fantasy, a quality or an experience.

Collage Messages
Each participant puts his/her name on an approximately 11" x 14" or larger piece of paper. On separate small pieces of paper, members write messages to one another. The messages are then glued to the appropriate person's paper.

Secret Friend
As in the traditional game, each participant chooses a name anonymously and leaves surprises for his/her secret friend.

Group Appreciation
The group forms a circle with the person receiving appreciation in the center.

Sufi Heart Dance
Participants form a circle. The Sufi Heart Dance done with soft music (such as Pachelbel) is a ritual movement to be done over and over. First, right arm down as an offering; then left arm down as an offering, lastly, lift your two hands together as receiving and place over your heart.

Pennies Activity
Each participant receives two pennies for making wishes. The group forms a circle with a penny pot in the center. Each participant makes one wish for him/herself, one wish for group.

Circle Form

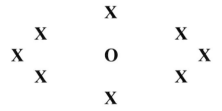

Person in the center receives appreciation from others and then without responding verbally, rejoins the group for the next person's turn.

Line Form

O

X

X

X

X

X

Each **X** gives feedback to **O**.
Then **O** goes to the end of the line and becomes an **X**.

One Word Sharing Cards
Each participant is given index cards equal to the number of other participants in the group. On each card, one for every other partici- pant, the person writes a word which s/he feel best describes that person. If there are twelve participants, each person will write eleven cards. Once this is completed, the participants exchange with each other the word that they have chosen for one another and a brief explanation of why they chose that word.

Medal of Honor
Names will be drawn and no one will know who has what name (until the end, if they choose). Each person will design a medal of honor for the person whose name s/he drew, making it as flashy as possible. On the medal will be written the person's name and a brief description of the quality of the person that it is honoring (e.g., "always considers the feelings of others," "makes people feel welcome in any group"). The medals will then be given out in a ceremony, presenting each person and his/her honor with great im- portance and putting the medal on him/her (pinning it or hanging it on a string around the neck), followed by applause from the group. Afterwards, solicit comments regarding how it felt to be honored or to have the spotlight on you.

Appreciation Gift

Put all participants' names in a hat. Each participant picks a name other than his/her own, and then creates an ornament or card for the person s/he picked. Have participants, as they give their gifts, share what they made for their chosen person, why and perhaps what they wish for that person or what they see as a positive quality, something that stands out about the person.

Wish

Divide the group in two and pick a volunteer facilitator for each group. The group facilitator writes down names of people in each group on pieces of paper then puts them in a container. Each person picks a name (not his/her own) and doesn't reveal the name that was picked. Each person draws a picture of what s/he wants the other person to have as a farewell present (about 5-10 minutes). Give the picture to the person.

Ceremonies for Change

All cultures have special ceremonies or rituals that celebrate changes in seasons, in government, or in individual status such as marriage or coming of age. Don't wait for a major event. Make a large or small change a reason to celebrate!

Planning your Celebration

- How do you want to celebrate?
- Will you celebrate privately — or do you want to involve others? A small or large group?
- Where and when will your celebration take place?
- How will you name or express the change? What personal symbols and symbolic actions will you use or create to illustrate the change and its positive effect on your life and therefore the lives of people you know?

- How will you begin your celebration? How will this set the tone for what will follow?
- Who do you want to be there? Will they take an active part in your celebration or be observers? Will you surprise them or will they help you plan the event?
- Will you speak spontaneously about your change or prepare remarks?
- Will you include any of the following? Songs, dance, music, poetry, stories, anecdotes, quotes, prayers, gifts, food, decorations, souvenirs, tributes?
- How will you connect your change to the power and love that exists in the world? How will you inspire your guests to make progress in their own lives?
- How will your ceremony end?
- Who's on the clean up committee?

5

Planning for the Creative Arts Group

In order for a program or group to be successful it is important to invest some time in planning. Time spent posing thoughtful questions and working out "glitches" in advance is time and energy that can be used for running the program rather than dealing with crises. Additionally, funding for programs is competitive and re-sources are not unlimited. Administrators are continually faced with demands for funds and support for a myriad of basic services, personnel and facilities. In order to give supervisors the confidence that resources for a creative arts group will be used wisely and suc-cessfully, it is important to propose a well-developed plan based on the anticipated or assessed needs of the clients.

Justifying a Creative Arts Group Program

Why should a particular facility support a creative arts pro-gram? What benefits will a creative arts group offer clients over another kind of group? These are questions the therapist should be able to answer, formally on paper or in his/her own mind, if s/he wants to institute a creative arts program in his/her setting. Being clear about why a proposed creative arts program benefits clients and enhances recreational therapy services helps communicate the program's value to supervisors, staff, clients and the public.

Benefits are the basis for explaining why a creative arts program is valuable to clients and the foundation for developing its goals. It may be helpful to gather information from journal articles and from books such as **Benefits of Therapeutic Recreation** (Coyle, Kinney, Riley & Shank, 1991). These provide information which can be given to supervisors about outcomes of creative arts programs. Benefits which may be mentioned include:

- Creativity is important to the developmental aspects of life. Creative arts influence the development of physical, cognitive, emotional, social and even vocational abilities.
- Creative arts encourage expression of thoughts and feelings in a tangible form that can be viewed by self and others. The creation of a product that is an extension of self can bring about insight, joy and/or feelings of self-esteem.
- Creative arts foster self-awareness and personal growth. Individuals experience a deepening understanding of themselves and their environment.
- By engaging the emotions, individuals are aided in moving to new levels of experience.
- Creative arts provide an opportunity to communicate both verbally and non-verbally, involving different thinking processes and abilities.

Space Considerations
for a Creative Arts Program

Ideally, a therapist should to be able to walk into a facility and have the perfect set up for doing creative arts, but that is not usually the case. Most therapists must adapt to their surroundings and make the available space work for them. The following are two suggestions for setting up a creative arts space that supports creative expression:

Size of Room(s).

If the facility has only one room to use for all creative arts (art, drama, movement, etc.) it should be a multipurpose or flexible space. It should be spacious enough for freedom of movement or relaxation but adaptable to more intimate work, such as writing or art. Some facilities have both an art room and a more general purpose room that can be used for exercise or more active movement. Some have a room with dividing walls that give the therapist the flexibility to change the space to suit his/her needs. Look at the room(s) available and determine what program(s) can be feasibly offered in that space.

Privacy.

No matter what kind of space is available at a facility, it needs to be private while the creative arts group meets. Freedom in creative expression comes from continuity of activity without distractions or interruptions.

Writing Goals

When interacting with clients, it is important to keep in mind the purpose of the group and what it should accomplish. Putting goals and objectives on paper helps clarify intentions before beginning to work with clients.

Goals are global statements of intent and lend direction to the program. The therapist should make sure that the goals for the program reflect the goals of his/her employer and the facility. Some sample goals that might be legitimately used in a creative arts program are

- to provide opportunities for wellness through creative self-expression.

- to enable clients to explore either individual problem areas and/or problems common to the group.

Objectives, particularly behavioral objectives, are specific statements which define the outcome or behavioral changes expected to occur as a result of the program. These objectives must be measurable, realistic and represent small, meaningful chunks of learning or change that the group can comfortably manage. An objective contains the conditions under which the behavior will take place, the criteria for knowing the client has achieved the desired behavior and the timeline for achievement. The following are sample behavioral objectives for a creative arts program:

- Client will attend to activity 5 (10, 20) minutes for 1 (2, 3) times per day.
- Client will maintain control and wait until staff is able to assist him/her in 50% (75%, 100%) of episodes.
- Client will tolerate activity 5 (10, 15) minutes without demonstrating anxious behavior 50% (75%, 100%) of the time.

Planning the Logistics

Logistics are the practical aspects of the program that must be addressed in order to enable it to operate smoothly. Forgetting to consider a logistic may mean that valuable time must later be spent trying to fix a problem that could have been avoided initially. Some logistical questions important to planning include:

- Where and when will the group meet?
- What is the starting date?
- What will be the length of the program?
- What is the most desirable size for the group? What are the minimum/maximum number of members allowable?
- How will clients learn about the group? PR — is there a facility newsletter, bulletin board, monthly calendar or community meeting to get the word out?

- How will clients get to the group? Is this well coordinated? If clients depend on staff to get them to this program, it is necessary to work with the staff to make sure this happens smoothly.
- What requirements are there for the area the group will use (accessible to wheelchair users, accessible to restrooms and drinking water)?
- What items are available at the facility (e.g., running water, tape player, chairs, pillows, tables)?
- What are the additional supplies needed for each meeting and throughout the program?
- Where can additional supplies be gotten and what are the costs (e.g., art materials, props such as hats, journals for writing)?
- Are adaptive devices needed (e.g., mouth apparatus for painting)?
- What are the emergency and fire safety plans? Are there first aid supplies? Who should be contacted in case of illness or injury?
- Will volunteers or assistants be present? What training needs to be done? Will we need to meet before or after sessions?

Checklist for a Creative Arts Group

The following is a checklist consisting of questions and considerations which can help in planning and assessing a creative arts program. Use it as a guideline, adding questions and categories as needed. The therapist should ask him/herself:

Leader Responsibilities and Considerations
- Who was I hired to be? A therapist? A play leader? A therapist specialist in drama, art, music, movement or dance?
- What are the strengths of my training?
- What are the limits of my training? (Be careful not to take on more responsibility than you are trained to handle.)

- What expectations of my supervisors am I supposed to meet? Are they realistic or do they need to be modified before the group begins?

Standards
- What (if any) city, county, state and/or federal regulations will I need to comply with?
- What (if any) voluntary standards (e.g., Joint Commission, CARF, American Camping Association) will I need to comply with?
- What facility/agency policies and procedures will I need to comply with?
- What professional standards will I need to comply with?
- What kind of documentation will I need to complete before, after each session? At the end of the program?

Before the group meets...
- What are the likely needs of this group?
- Written plan with goals for the group: Particularly in the case of a new program but also if you are a new facilitator to an existing group, it is helpful to think out your plan on paper. Some settings have a planning form but, if none exists, the proposal should include the name of the group, what is to be accomplished (the goals), how logistics will be dealt with and information on how the program will be evaluated.
- What are the strengths and limitations of the place where we will be meeting and of the resources available to me?

Who is in the group?
- Do I have all the information I need about group members? Do I have some sense of who each person is as well as the composition of the entire group?

- Do I know the diagnoses listed for group members — including the definition, impact on functional ability and precautions to take?
- Is this a voluntary or mandatory group?
- Is membership in the group fluid? Can members "drop in?"
- Is this a newly formed group? If not, how can I find out the past history of the group?
- Do group members know one another from another setting?
- What might be the cohesive factor in the group? Is it a group for women, teens, veterans?

Planning the Sessions
- What are the objectives for sessions?
- What kind of behavior is anticipated/desired for each session?
- How much structure does the group need? Does the group need a more directive style of leadership (leader more authoritative in giving specific directions) or a more facilitative leadership approach (leader trying to include more client ideas to set direction)?
- What activities are most appropriate to the needs and potential of the group? It may be helpful to use some aspect of the activity analysis process if unsure of whether or not an activity will have the desired outcome. Activity analysis is the systematic application of a set of variables used to break down and examine a given activity for the purpose of understanding its inherent qualities, participation factors or outcome possibilities.
- Do I have good resources for activities or know where to find them or someone who might help brainstorm ideas?
- Can the activities that have been planned be modified to meet individual situations which may arise during the group?
- Do I have specific ideas of what I will be looking for as I observe the group?
- Do I have a budget and a detailed list of materials and supplies which need to be purchased?

During the Session

- For new groups — introductions of members and leader. Discuss what the group will be doing. Discuss rules, agreements and mandatory behavior. Encourage group suggestions and reactions.
- What warm-up activity/activities will be used?
- What is the general mood of the group? What criteria will be used to assess this? (e.g., Will I ask a question at the beginning of each group or do the same song or activity each time and observe the group's energy and response?)
- What are some of the groups concerns and goals — as a whole? As individuals?
- Does the process seem interesting? If the answer is no, probably no one else is challenged either.

Post-Session Evaluation

- How did it go? What happened that was unexpected? Positive? Negative?
- What was the group response to the therapist, helpers, the material, to each other?
- Did the goals and objectives seem appropriate and productive? Were they achieved?
- Should there be new goals and objectives for the group, for individual members?
- Record observations in a journal or in individual charts. Be sure to meet documentation requirements of employer, professional and accrediting agencies.

Planning for the Next Session

- Do I want the group to continue in the same basic direction?
- Are there changes I want to make in approach, use of time and area, degree of supervision or explanation, degree of intervention?
- Are individual members being well served?

- Compare your initial, pre-meeting impressions and perceptions of the group members with those you have now. What insights does this give you about yourself as the group's leader and about the group itself?

Modification of Experiences

Our job as therapists is to create opportunities for individuals to participate in our programs as fully as possible. We have to be flexible in our thinking and willing to modify a program as needed. Sometimes a formerly successful activity will not work with a new group and needs revision. The following guidelines (taken from **Closing the Gap**, by the Department of Recreation and Leisure Studies at San Jose State University, 1989) are basic considerations to keep in mind to help modify your program, if needed:

1. Think *abilities*. Base modifications on what participants can do. For example, if some members have limited vision, consider their abilities to hear, smell and touch. Add auditory and tactile clues to a visual experience to enable everyone to participate. Everyone's experience will be broadened.

2. Take your *cues* from participants. For example, never remove crutches from a person when that person is seated, unless a request is made. Wheelchairs, artificial limbs, crutches, canes and walkers are part of what the person needs to function as fully as possible. There are enough challenges without creating unnecessary ones. If one of your participants falls down, do not panic or rush over like a paramedic. The person will let you know if and how much assistance is needed, and how to do it. Common sense and preservation of dignity must combine to create a good solution. With time, everyone will read each other's cues accurately, and routines will be worked out for dealing with various situations.

3. Change a *location* if necessary to minimize the limitations of environmental barriers. Think of the surface you will be using

if there are participants who use wheelchairs. A harder surface is easier to maneuver on than a soft one. Anticipate potential barriers. Always verify wheelchair access. File appropriate complaints if access is not provide where the law requires it.

4. *Preserve* the experience and its components as close to the original activity as you possibly can. Modify only those elements that need to be adapted. In this way the skills learned in this environment will be more easily applied to situations at school, work, at the park or the world at large.

5. *Involve* those who know — your clients — in the adaptation process. This not only encourages them to create their own leisure experiences outside the group but they often have ideas about what would be useful. They often know or have heard of something that works well. They will also reap the good feelings of finding alternatives for others are well as themselves.

6. *Learn* everything you can about adaptive and special equipment that help participants with physical disabilities participate fully in daily living. Try to make adaptive equipment available to include an individual in an experience. Become an advocate for inclusion of these items in the budget of your facility.

7. *Create* and introduce new experiences in order to encourage group cohesion, build self-confidence and widen participants' interests. Occasionally these experiences can require that all participants experience a limitation in common. For example, games can be planned in the dark or with blindfolds. Another possibility is to instruct the participants to communicate only through non-verbal use of their face and body from the waist up. They will gain a new perspective on gestures, facial expressions, drawing, writing, for example. In this as well as other activities, adaptations must be individualized whenever possible.

8. The Bottom Line. Ask yourself these questions as you modify the activities for your participants. Your answers are *critical factors* in the decisions you make. If you find that you are not thrilled with some of the answers you give, take up the chal-

lenge to overcome your limitations as you work to make life fuller and more inclusive for others:

- Are you overprotective and too ready to jump in? Do you become so anxious that you don't give a participant the "extra" time and effort to do something without assistance?
- Do you wait until your assistance is requested?
- Do your assumptions limit your participants before you have really had a chance to get to fully know them and their situations?
- Is your idea of a successful activity realistic and optimistic at the same time?
- Do you focus on a person's eyes and general presence rather than the wheelchair or other indicator of disability?
- Is one of your goals to sometimes forget that the person has a disability?

Multicultural and Lifestyle Choice Considerations

We live in a social environment that is increasingly complex and culturally diverse. As a therapist you will probably be working with people whose first language is not English and/or whose life experiences, values, norms and family support systems may be different from your own. What it requires from you is a more honest and astute level of consciousness. Just as people make suppositions about individuals with disabilities they also make subconscious judgments about people whose lives and histories are different from their own. Some suggestions to help you be not just "politically correct" but more importantly "humanly conscious" in your attitudes and interactions:

- Remember that all of us are products of culture. We have values, attitudes and ways of dealing with situations that we learned through our families and support systems. Respect the differences between people and help others look for commonalties.

- Be aware of subliminal assumptions on your part or others. Treat everyone as an individual, not as a member of a subgroup. Get to know how that individual thinks, feels and lives.
- Creative arts have the capacity to overcome differences in language, background, abilities and experiences. Music, dance and art speak to all of us without the need for one language. Celebrate multicultural richness by choosing activities from different cultures to use in the group.

People Resources and Supportive Funding

These days, many facilities have just enough staff to get by. In many situations it is appropriate to have volunteers that can help clients get set up and can assist clients as needed. A successful volunteer program takes organization, thought, time and good public relations. Do not initiate a volunteer program if staff are too busy to listen to volunteers' concerns or provide needed training. A good volunteer program, once created, can enhance the quality of a therapist's individual contact with clients. Some reminders about successful supervision:

- Think about what kind of help will be needed. Make sure that you are clear about the tasks you want your volunteer to complete. Take the time to write a job description for the volunteer(s).
- Create a scrapbook of photos, artwork, and background information about the program or develop a volunteer handbook. Take these recruitment materials to college classes or community organizations so that interested people can get a better feel about the nature of the program.
- Structure a training process for volunteers to introduce them to the agency, clients and their duties. Make sure you have the right person doing the right kind of job.

- For volunteers completing college fieldwork, be clear about the requirements (e.g., amount of hours, nature of client contact) and make sure that the contract is being upheld.
- Listen to and observe volunteers in order to assess how their experiences are proceeding and make adjustments before problems arise.
- Don't think of volunteers as "fill-in help." Treat them with respect, reward them with praise or other benefits and write thoughtful letters of recommendation if asked.

Whenever volunteer or financial support is needed, it is important to know where to find the appropriate resources. The following are ideas to help start the search:

Fieldwork and Internships for Colleges and Universities

Many students must complete fieldwork hours to graduate in their major. Check with professional schools such as education, recreational therapy, occupational therapy, social work, psychology, art or other media to find out if they require fieldwork hours. A responsible student brings fresh energy and ideas to the program. Additionally, if directed properly, a college student who has a fieldwork requirement will be available on a regular basis for at least a semester's time.

Volunteer Bureau

A community volunteer bureau sees many people in the course of a day and might be able to locate a retired artist, music teacher, dance instructor or even an art lover who might be a valuable volunteer. Make sure the volunteer bureau has a clear job description of the position so they can refer the right person to the program.

Personal Resources

If you are comfortable with these activities, public speaking and/or writing can augment other funding.

Community Organizations

Some organizations will donate time or money to help a program in their community. For example, if the facility is having a special hands-on arts program for children with disabilities, it may be possible to approach local organizations and ask them to sponsor some aspect of the program. This involves some time and energy in making presentations and coordinating funding, but is the kind of involvement that benefits everyone.

Corporate Funding or Arts Support

Many corporations create philanthropic foundations which often focus on supporting programs in their own communities or counties. Some corporations will exhibit art in their buildings — they get some lovely art for their walls and good public relations and the arts group receives a space to exhibit and public awareness for the program. The University of Maryland Library has an excellent web page for locating information on these grants (Grants and Awards in the Visual Arts: Sources of Information: http://www.lib.umd.edu/UMCP/ART/guides/grants.htm).

Government Funding for the Arts

Arts funding trickles down from the federal level to state, county and city. Each state receives funding for arts programming which is distributed through the arts councils (counties and city commissions) in that state. Check for the kinds of programs that are being funded by local arts councils. Some county arts councils, for example, will fund artists to teach their craft to clients in community nonprofit organizations.

"Very Special Arts"

Very Special Arts is an international organization that supports art programs serving individuals with disabilities. Since 1974, **Very Special Arts** has created opportunities primarily for children with disabilities in dance, drama, music, literature and visual arts. These children and young adults have participated in a variety of **Very Special Arts** activities, including festivals, school programs, special projects, performances and exhibitions. You can reach them at 1300 Connecticut Ave., Washington, DC 20036. Phone: 800-933-8721, e-mail: info@vsarts.org.

Planning for the Visual Arts Group

Up to this point the planning ideas for arts groups have been very general and could be applied to any type of group. This last section addresses concerns of special interest to the therapist setting up a visual arts group and deals with materials, space considerations, and tips and techniques for client populations with specific disabilities or health concerns.

A Space for Art

Most facilities do not come equipped with the "Cadillac" of art spaces; most therapists will have to make do with a "rebuilt Volkswagen." The following are basic necessities for the room to be used as an art space:

- adequate lighting — for all individuals but especially for those with visual impairments.
- ready access to a sink and water.
- an area adequate for the group, with enough table space and chairs to accommodate everyone comfortably. Do your best with this requirement given the limits of your facility.
- storage space (locked) — enough space to enable good organization of materials for easy access.

- good ventilation — some people (especially those with respiratory problems) are very sensitive to chemicals in paint. Make sure to keep air circulating through the space.
- capability for privacy — if involved in an art therapy technique or an activity that involves guided imagery it will be necessary to block out exterior distractions.
- display area — at times it is appropriate to display some of the art created by clients. Make sure there is at least a bulletin board for this purpose.

Materials of Art

Art materials can be expensive. The key is to be smart about how to stretch the budget and resourceful in finding materials that can be gathered cheaply. Many people who lead art groups are pack rats by nature. They see rejected stuff as potential material for art. Students in our classes have brainstormed in groups about items to save from around the house to use in visual art projects and amazingly the list has kept growing every year.

Materials to Spend Money On

If the program does have a budget, considering spending some of the money on these items:

- **Paint brushes.** It is a waste of money to buy cheap brushes. After limited use the hairs often come out and the brush loses its shape. There are great brushes now for smaller children that have flexible brush tips but durable, easy to hold handles that will take a lot of beating from small children. If you are working with adolescents or adults, it is important to have a variety of sizes in brushes and tip shapes (e.g., flat or round) for satisfying results. Build up a supply slowly, if necessary, and teach clients how to clean and store the brushes properly.

- **Scissors.** Nothing is more frustrating than scissors that don't cut properly. Buy good, sturdy scissors that are appropriate for the age of the clients and if possible have some scissors for people who are left-handed — they'll be deeply appreciated.

- **Paper.** There are a wide range of papers and uses to be considered:
  - *butcher paper* — Purchase a large roll of butcher paper that will cover general use and casual scribbling.
  - *recycled computer paper, old stationery and leftover posters* — for scribbling and idea building.
  - *newsprint* — good for pencil and charcoal work, some can take a little wet media.
  - *construction* paper — try to get a non-fading variety, if possible. Scraps can be recycled for collage and other uses.
  - *drawing* papers — Some varieties can also handle ink, markers or watercolor. Get the most diversity out of the paper.
  - *tracing* paper — you can work out a drawing on tracing paper and transfer it to good paper without damaging the surface of the good paper by erasing and reworking on it.
  - *fancy* paper — for watercolor or acrylic painting. Use a weight of paper that can handle some working, at least 60 pounds.
  - *handmade* paper — beautiful paper can be created using a blender, paper scraps of all sorts and even leaves. These papers can be used for painting and collage and are all the more special because they are handmade.

- **Paints.** Keep a supply of basic tempera paints available in plastic jars. If working with children, buy containers with color coded tops and snappable, non-spill lids to keep paint in for ready use. If cake watercolor is used, buy the kind that can give you more variety in value (i.e., lightness or darkness of color).

Some only give you pale color. Markers are fun (as long as the tops get put back on!) — children love the scented ones. For older children or adults, add things like chalk or oil pastel. Oil pastels are a great alternative to oil paint — they are less messy and can be blended with turpentine for interesting effects. Acrylics, watercolors or oil paints in tubes are expensive — look for student grade supplies. They are a bit cheaper and fine for group artwork.

Being Resourceful

Packrats will be in heaven when they read this list of things to save from around the house for art projects. The only limitation is storage area, but this can usually be cleverly organized as well.

Materials to Save

- alphabet soup letters
- baby food jars
- bag twisties
- beads (old necklaces from thrift stores/flea market)
- beans (dried)
- bottle caps
- boxes (little to as big as you can store)
- broken crayons
- broken toys
- buttons
- calendars (for photos or pictures)
- cardboard scraps (corrugated and other interesting surfaces)
- chop sticks (great for scooping paint or mixing materials)
- coffee cans
- computer paper (quick, casual drawings)
- corks
- cotton balls
- dried flowers
- egg cartons (for paints, sorting of beads/sequins)
- fabric scraps (for collage, masks)
- game pieces from old games
- gloves (for puppets)
- ice trays (palette)
- jars (all sizes for storage)

- magazines (for collage, ideas for topics)
- margarine containers (for storage)
- newspaper
- noodles and other pasta (for collage)
- oatmeal boxes
- old jewelry (for masks, collage, puppets)
- old socks (for puppets)
- paper bags (for masks, puppets)
- plastic bubble packing material (for collage)
- polished glass or rock from beach (for masks, sculpture)
- rags (for cleaning)
- rocks and twigs (for masks, sculpture, collage)
- rubber bands
- salt (for use in recipes for sculpture materials)
- shoe boxes
- string
- Styrofoam (for collage)
- tiles (for sculpture)
- tissue paper and wrapping paper scraps
- wallpaper scraps
- wood scraps (for sculpture)
- yarn and ribbon ends (for collage, puppets)

Where to Find Resources

Most communities are gold mines for leftover materials that can be recycled as art. Brainstorm a list of places to check for help in stocking the art area. Some ideas that have been contributed by our students:

- appliance stores (for very large boxes that can be used for sculpture)
- plastics stores that sell plastic tubing and sheeting may allow rummaging through their remnants for sculpture supplies
- garage sales (for beads and other reusable items)
- lumber yards (for wood scraps)
- fabric stores (for throw-away scraps and remnants)
- cardboard or packing companies (will donate unusable remnants)

The community might even have an art recycling center where manufacturers can donate materials for use by non-profit agencies for a minimal fee.

Being creative about collecting resources is both fun and wise. Money saved in one area means being able to obtain a greater quantity or better quality of materials (like brushes) that must be bought.

Compensatory Techniques and Useful Tips

There are a number of compensatory techniques which can help clients with disabilities participate more fully and successfully in artistic experiences. Specific adaptive devices are also available (generally through catalogs) to assist clients who would benefit from a modified technique.

General Techniques

- Use masking tape to fasten paper, fabric, cardboard or other flat items to the worktable.
- Attach suction cups to the bottoms of plates, cups, jars and bottles to be decorated. Suction cups are also useful for bottoms of paint jars to prevent knocking over and spilling. Especially useful are suction soap holders, modeling clay or floral putty. The non-slip pads used under throw rugs also work well when they are cut to size.
- Build up the handles of tools and utensils such as paint brushes, screwdrivers, utility knives or crochet hooks by wrapping sponge or foam rubber around the handle until it is a comfortable width. Tape the foam firmly into place. Tape the end of the foam to the tool handle to avoid slipping.
- Build up the arm of a chair to a comfortable working height by taping foam or folded towels to the top of the chair arm. The

problem of a hand tremor may be reduced to a minimum when the elbow is supported on the chair arm.

- To assist someone with limited motor control to cut paper or fabric, insert the paper or stiff fabric into the center of a thick book and cut with bent-handled scissors.
- Avoid skin abrasion by attaching sandpaper to smooth blocks of wood with tacks, or use sanding blocks available in hardware and paint stores.
- Use "C" clamps to fasten looms, stretcher frames or weaving frames to the worktable, holding the frame in a convenient, upright position.
- Hold work for sewing by attaching one edge of the work to a table with masking tape and weighting down the work in the lap with a book or other suitable object.

Tips for People with Limited Vision

- Work with bright colors. Neutral, pastel or subtle colors are frequently difficult to identify or differentiate.
- Use thick yarns, large-eyed needles, larger beads. Think bigger to reduce frustration in working on projects.
- In painting or drawing with color, think of creating simple patterns with large areas of color and little detail. Rather than detail, work with shape, color, texture. These alone can create interesting pieces of art. Abstracts are particularly suitable.
- Investigate the market of assorted aids such as magnifiers that clip onto eyeglasses, magnifiers on stands, magnifiers worn around the neck. Consult a physician as to the suitability of any of these aids for a particular individual.
- Develop the sense of touch by experimenting with arts or crafts that are particularly suited to people with vision problems: working with clay, weaving and mosaic tile work are examples.

Tips for People with Arthritis

- Electric scissors are easier to use than hand scissors.
- Macramé, rug hooking, weaving and working with clay are particularly good exercises for the fingers.
- Knitting and crocheting should be avoided because the fingers are held stiffly for long periods of time.
- Handles of tools can be built up to avoid the necessity of holding the fingers in a tight grasp.

Tips for People with Sensitive Skin

- Use plastic gloves, preferably the thin disposable surgical type, for any messy work. (Be careful of latex sensitivity, though.)
- Ask clients if there are any materials which cause reactions and avoid them or use substitutes whenever possible.
- Use acrylic yarns instead of wool.
- Avoid handling abrasives such as sandpaper. Mount sandpaper on a wood block or in a plastic holder to keep away from skin.
- Keep hand cream available and use it to keep the skin as supple as possible.

Tips for People with Respiratory Problems

- Work in a well-ventilated room. It is possible to purchase excellent air filters that are quiet and very effective in maintaining a high quality of air in the room.
- Use water-based paints and adhesives that have no objectionable odors or harmful fumes. The brushes, sponges and cloths for these products are cleaned in water, thus eliminating the use of harmful thinners such as turpentine.
- Avoid projects involving sanding unless you can work outdoors or in a room with an exhaust fan. Use a mask as added protection against inhaling dust.
- Avoid all aerosol products.

- Work positions which allow the head to be held up and the shoulders back, allow for good air exchange. Hunched over postures reduce lung capacity.

Tips for People with Short Attention Spans

- Reduce stimulus in the work space.
- Limit the variety of tool and supply options available at any given time.
- Have the clients sit *around* a table so that their attention is always focused inward (toward the center of the table) and not around the room.
- If possible, put the light source directly over the table leaving the walls of the room dimmer.
- Soothing music, with little variation in the melody, may help.
- A fan in the background may produce enough "white noise" to mask other, more distracting background noise.

6

Visual and Tactile Arts

This chapter provides an overview of concepts relating to art and art therapy and offers activity ideas for using visual arts with clients. The term "visual and tactile arts" refers to a product or process that uses art materials to create a form that can be experienced by seeing or touching. This area can demand a lot of a therapist's time and budget in procuring and organizing materials, but it has the capacity to engage clients from a wide range of ages and backgrounds. Most people who have gone through the school system have had some exposure to art and have some association that helps them connect to the topic when it is introduced. Some clients may have had more positive experiences in art than others but at least there is some basis for communication with most individuals.

Helping clients learn about themselves from these art activities involves several stages of processing. First there is the pure *doing* of the activity, which uses both the conscious thinking mind and the unconscious expressive mind. Once the activity is completed, it is important to help clients decipher and digest what *they* have experienced. This is achieved by having clients answer questions or reflect on some part of the art activity using writing. Writing uses symbols (left brain) to communicate ideas and helps bring the ideas into one's consciousness. Finally, clients are invited to share what happened or what they learned with a partner or the group as a whole. The expression of ideas in words clarifies the individual's thoughts and allows other group members to give feedback and provide more insight for the individual. It is the therapist's job to do whatever s/he can to make the learning "real" and to cement a helpful concept in the mind of the client so it has a chance to incubate and grow.

Types of Visual Arts Experiences

In visual arts there are a range of expressions that classify the activities, with each activity having its own purpose.

Fine Arts
Traditionally this refers to art (e.g., painting, drawing, sculpture) that focuses on the aesthetic (pure beauty) and is created for its own sake. The individual expresses his/her own views and feelings about a subject and takes pleasure in using the materials to create a form that can be experienced by the artist and others. The process of creating the art may have therapeutic value to the artist but this is not a goal for fine arts.

Crafts
This refers to art (e.g., weaving, jewelry making, ceramics) that is produced for utilitarian purposes. The artist is making something pleasing to be used by people in their homes and in their lives.

Therapeutic Art
This refers to art therapy or techniques used in therapeutic interventions. In this realm the focus is on *process* rather than on product and the therapist is a facilitator of experiences that can lead to increased psychological well being.

While these categories help to differentiate functions of art, there are many examples of overlapping categories that help us to view them more flexibly. For example, a mask created for a therapeutic purpose may have beauty and capture the essence of human experience — it can be also thought of as fine art. Or an individual engaged in making a craft may experience feelings of well being and calm that could be attributed to therapeutic art.

Skills Involved in Art Activities

Clients are likely to be receiving a therapist's services because they are having problems and are functioning below their optimum level. While engaging in creative arts activities may enhance clients' functional skills and quality of life, asking them to become involved in activities that are beyond their abilities may actually cause harm. The art activities suggested in this chapter assume that clients have a certain skill set. This checklist should be consulted if there is any doubt about the ability of a group member to participate in art activities in general or in using a particular medium.

General Skills

- Some degree of muscle and hand-eye coordination
- Reasonable endurance for starting and engaging in activity
- Tolerance and willingness to touch clay and other supplies which make one "dirty" (not tactilely defensive)
- Basic problem solving skills
- Ability to follow one, two or three step instructions
- Ability to function independently in a semi-structured environment
- Basic communication and listening skills
- Willingness to relate to others
- Basic social skills
- Capacity to deal with emotions evoked by activities

Uses of Art Materials in Therapeutic Situations

Art materials can be used by the therapist to refine *behavior* as well as to encourage expression and enhance learning. As the therapist develops his/her treatment goals for a group, s/he will need to make sure that the art medium complements the desired goals. Some art media encourage active, expressive movements, while other media encourage expression within very specific limits.

Some of these materials overlap categories, being (for instance) both compulsive and expressive in nature. However, if one considers the psychological issues involved in doing a particular project, each type may be clearly considered for a specific purpose or goal. In addition to using these materials, there is always the invitation and encouragement to draw — drawing *feelings* rather than objects.

Compulsive Art Materials

Restrictive, limiting boundaries can be ego supporting and help enhance impulse control through sublimation.

- Sticks, wood
- weavings
- monoprints, stencils, rubbings
- pencils with rulers
- mosaics
- manipulating geometric forms

Regressive Art Materials

Can lead to regression due to inability to find or control boundaries, psychological and/or concrete. Can be very satisfying if able to use.

- water colors
- finger paints
- clay (has no form)

Aggressive Art Materials

Allow for expression of aggression, which can be used to elicit repressed feelings or as a way of sublimating the action of aggression.

- torn paper collage
- splatter painting
- wood and nails

Expressive Art Materials

Allow for non-verbal expression of thoughts, feelings and ideas.

- crayon
- crayon resist
- string painting
- cut photo paper
- wood sculptures
- collage
- body outline
- paper masks
- puppets
- brush painting
- felt tip pen
- chalk
- mobiles
- pencil

Activities Grouped by Type of Medium

This section first examines drawing and painting as therapeutic activities and then discusses the therapeutic uses of clay.

Drawing and Painting as Therapeutic Activities

Many of the activities offered in this chapter are done using some method of painting or drawing. It is helpful to focus further on drawing and painting as valuable therapeutic processes which promote self-awareness and expression.

Drawing

A line can be a powerful and evocative tool for the individual exploring expression. A dark, heavy line could express sadness; a pale, delicate line could communicate fragility or insecurity. Through drawing, the client uses line, color, shape and texture to help express existing feelings that are difficult to verbalize and communicate.

Have larger sheets of paper (at least 18" x 24") available so that group members can feel more expansive by using more of their bodies in drawing. For media use colored pencils, felt tip pens, crayons, charcoal or pastels. In using painting or drawing have participant(s) answer open ended questions such as, "How do I feel at this moment?" or "Where am I right now in my life?"

Painting

Making strokes, shapes and textures on paper using a brush and paint can give clients a feeling of movement and fluidity. It is especially helpful to a client who is blocked in terms of feeling and/or expression. When working on opening blocked expression, it is helpful to have clients paint standing up using a large piece of paper taped on the wall. This enables them to see more clearly what they are doing, to use more of their body in the painting process, to feel freedom of movement and perhaps tap into emotions that are locked up in parts of the body. Have them warm-up by painting for 5 minutes, then 10 minutes and finally give them a time frame for a longer piece of work. In the beginning, clients will need help structuring the time they spend on each painting. The goal is for the clients to eventually become sensitive to when they think their paintings are finished.

Painting and Drawing Activities

Drawing Objects Game (a version of Pictionary)
Players are divided into two teams. Each has a stack of paper and pencils at equal distance from the leader. Group leader has a list of objects (like a Christmas tree or a house) and persons (like a cook or fireman) which have distinguishing characteristics. One player from each team comes to the leader in the center. The leader tells the two players one object to draw. Each member runs back to

his/her team and draws it. The first member on a team to correctly guess the object or person being drawn wins. Remind groups that no talking is allowed.

Picture Mosaic and Enlargement

Choose a photograph or a picture from a magazine that is colorful and interesting. Cut it up into equally sized squares and on the back make an identification so you will know the how to reassemble the pieces. Show the entire picture to the group briefly. Then, give each group member or pair of participants a piece of the picture and a larger piece of paper to depict and enlarge their part. The goal is to recreate the essence of their part of the picture. It does not need to be a duplication. At the end, reassemble the parts and glue them to a large sheet of cardboard.

Combining Art and Music

Butcher paper with a large circle drawn in the middle is laid out on the floor. Each group member makes a picture of an animal with its tail inside the center circle. To play, the leader steps on tails (can also be developed as a storytelling process) and when a particular tail is stepped on the designated participant makes the animal sound or another note until the leader releases the tail.

Symphony of Emotions on Paper

Participants are asked how they feel and to express this on paper with crayons, markers or paint. Then, each person is asked to produce a sound representative of their emotion. When their picture is touched by leader, they make their sound. The leader conducts a symphony of emotions. Everyone must pay attention and begin and end exactly on cue.

Group Mural

Each person picks one colored crayon or magic marker and decides on one shape to draw (examples: lines, dots, circles, squiggles) during the entire activity. One long, continuous piece of paper is spread out on a table or the floor. People line up on all sides of the paper and draw their shapes on one section of the paper for approximately one minute. The leader says "switch" and each person moves to a new section and draws his/her shape again. The activity is repeated until the mural is completed.

Mural of a Town

Attach a large sheet of butcher paper to a wall with masking tape. Provide a variety of materials: paints, crayons, felt tip pens as well as scissors, glue and tactile objects (e.g., yarn, crepe paper) if desired. The group, through discussion and compromise, designs a town. A basic outline is agreed upon. Then each person chooses a different part of the town such as a building or park to work on. Each individual will need to look at his/her own needs for food, clothing, safety, entertainment, for example, in deciding what form the town will take. Suggest that individuals check with their potential neighbors (i.e., other group members) and make necessary accommodations to each other's needs. When the mural is completed, the group can discuss how they feel about their town.

Initials

Provide sheets of paper, pencils, felt tip markers and crayons. Each participant draws his/her own initials in any style, size or color s/he wishes. The initials may be plain or elaborate, large or small depending one what individuals wish to share about themselves with other members of the group. Clients are invited to share their completed drawings and talk about them, if they want to.

Drawing Pass

Each client will have one piece of paper and will be asked to draw a few lines on it and sign it. The paper is next passed to the right and each person adds to the previous drawing. This sequence is repeated until the paper is returned to its original creator. The results can be shared or not and comments solicited as to thoughts and feelings about the task.

The Therapeutic Value of Clay

Working with earth is one of our earliest artistic experiences. As children, many of us made mud pies and even whole mud villages. If you close your eyes and remember the cool, smooth feel of earth, you will understand why clay is an appealing and therapeutic modality. Earth is one of the traditional four elements and is an ancient icon of nature, growth and mother in human experience and thought.

Working with clay has a calming influence on many clients, especially if the initial focus of the work is on process rather than product. As clients become more familiar with the medium, the results of their work can be striking.

Objectives
- To become comfortable with and sensitive to the medium of clay through tactile exploration.
- To allow for the release of tension and expression of feelings through clay.
- To provide for the use of clay as a bridge for interaction with other people.

Clay Activities

As with a blank piece of paper, a lump of clay can be very intimidating to clients. It takes a while for people to learn how to work the clay and to create a shape that communicates an idea or feeling. When clients first look at the clay they will be drawn to "make something" out of the lump of earth in front of them. Try to de-emphasize this desire to create something representational by focusing on process rather than product. By taking the time to explore the clay a client can experience the almost meditative and calming value of working with clay.

How willing clients are to enjoy the journey (process) rather than the destination (product) is valuable information for each individual.

Clay Exploration (Warm-ups)

- Provide enough clay for each individual and also water and sponges for clean-up.
- Have each person take a piece of clay. Encourage exploring the properties of the clay: Is it wet, cold, elastic? Suggest that group members knead, stretch, flatten, tear, squeeze and poke holes through clay. Optional materials: rolling pins, shaping tools and fabrics (e.g., lace) that will transfer texture to the clay
- Ask group members to create a shape with their clay that shows how they are feeling. The form may be abstract or representational.
- Allow group members to talk about their shape if they wish. This activity encourages self-expression and gives the therapist a clue to each person's emotional state.

Create a Fantasy Creature

Ask participants to imagine themselves as a creature and make that creature with the clay. Encourage each person to describe his/her creature or have it "speak" to the group. Ask each person to be his/her creature and introduce him/herself as "I am...," and/or to speak about what it's like to be that creature.

Variation: Ask group members to imagine themselves as an object or symbol (e.g., star, tree, mountain) and create that image in clay. Continue as above by having each person in the group introduce him/herself, for example, "I am the star burning inside, too hot to get close to..."

Create in Pairs

Divide group into pairs. Ask the partners to create something together. It can be a place they would like to be or something fun they would like to do together. Ask them to include themselves in the sculpture.

Self Portrait in Clay

Instruct group members to make their self portrait in sculpture. Ask participants to depict themselves as they believe they really are, which includes their feelings/current state of being. For example, if anger is a dominate emotion, the sculpture should reflect this emotion. Group members can also depict how they would like to be/feel. Discussion of the activity should deal with the differences between these images and what actions might help them reach a more desirable state of being.

Activities Grouped by Therapeutic Outcome

These techniques come from art therapists who use a variety of them, depending on the required outcomes for their clients. The six categories, developed by art therapist James Denny (1972), are classified according to the expected kinds of effect experienced by the participant. Depending on the stage of the group's development, some activities will be more or less challenging to introduce to the members. For example, a therapist wouldn't use an activity like "self-portrait" with a new group but rather something in the area of exploration of media. Each of the six categories is described and has suggested, identifiable behavioral goals.

I. Exploration

Exploration activities are especially useful in the initial sessions of a group when the therapist is trying to introduce clients to the art experience. Many therapists will continue to use exploratory exercises throughout the sessions, sometimes as warm-up or closure activities. These activities are similar to free association and encourage spontaneous expression. Since they focus not on product but on process, they help release conscious controls on expression. The techniques are simple, direct and liberating.

Behavioral Goals:
Participants will:

- Express themselves spontaneously by drawing on paper with various art media.
- Become acquainted (or reacquainted) with art materials by using four different types of media in some way.
- Explore the use of these media in making lines, symbols and forms, and by making a design using at least two different media.

Scribble Drawings
Have clients do these with eyes open and/or shut. Be sensitive to the group and how much time they are comfortable doing this kind of open-ended activity. For a number of these free form activities, start with one minute and gradually build up to more time.

Finger Painting
For adults this can be a regressive kind of experience and can evoke memories of childhood. It is a kind of scribbling that uses more of the body. Slick finger painting paper can be purchased to ease the experience and flow of finger-painting.

Free Drawings
The subject and the media are choices left to the client. "Free" (spontaneous) expression is encouraged; "planning the picture" is discouraged. Initially, free drawing should be done for one to two minutes, after which the amount of time can be gradually increased. Encourage clients to maintain an "empty mind" and not preconceive stories or images.

Ink Blot
Using watercolors or ink, create a blob of color on the paper. The paper may then be folded (by client or therapist) like a Rorschach. Write a story or make a statement about the image on the paper.

Straw Painting
Place a blob of liquid color on paper and gently blow on the color with a straw. The end result might suggest an image or evoke a thought or feeling.

Build a Curiosity Picture
Write two letters (e.g., G and H) on a piece of paper. Use crayons, markers or oil pastels to create an abstract design out of the letters by connecting lines, filling spaces, putting in squiggles and/or by any other means. Many clients are intimidated by a blank sheet of paper — having something already on the paper can help motivate the client (Landgarten, 1981).

Watercolor/Crayon Resist
This activity encourages exploration of flow and resistance effects. Crayon is used to make designs on paper, then water color paints are applied. The crayon "resists" the flow of the watercolors, creating interesting patterns.

Clay
It is especially helpful when introducing clay to an inexperienced group to start at stage one — exploration. This means experiencing the "feel" of the clay — its texture and movement possibilities. The clients should be encouraged to roll and pound the clay, to form and crumble shapes. Helps to acquaint clients with how the medium works.

Edible Art
This technique is especially good with children or individuals with visual challenges. Introduce finger-painting with pudding or icing with food coloring, incorporating the senses of taste, smell and touch. Sculpture can be made with oatmeal or bread dough. Print-making can be done with vegetables and fruits.

Automatic Drawing
Good for bypassing the critical mind that wants everything to look "right." Some ideas:
- Make free lines or scribbles on paper first with eyes open and then with eyes closed.
- Draw using the non-dominant hand.
- Draw by not taking the hand off the paper until the picture is complete.

Media and Color Exploration
- Make blobs and dribbles on wet paper with watercolor.
- Make blobs and dribbles on paper with ink.
- Make a non-representational, free form design with pastels or crayons.
- Make a design using two different types of media.

II. Rapport Building

This level is designed to facilitate a more natural transition between creation and exploration. The techniques help prepare the individual to express ideas and feelings from the self by conceptualizing and sharing ideas with another person and creating something with the support of a group member. Other objectives of rapport building are to encourage exchanges between participants and support development of a group identity.

Pair Scribble
Members form pairs, each has his/her own drawing tool but they share a piece of paper. They are not to speak but to somehow work together to fill the page during a period of 3-5 minutes. What occurs depends on the personalities of the group. The "natural leaders" lead, the followers tend to follow, and the negotiators work out compromise and cooperation. This activity reveals one's unconscious style of doing things.

Variation: Scribble and Completion. One person makes a scribble and the other person converts the scribble into an image or builds upon the scribble in some way.

Pictionary
The game of Pictionary™, which involves guessing a word or phase from an image drawn on paper, is a good way to introduce playfulness into the art process. The game also helps people address the fear of drawing images on a blank piece of paper.

Non-Verbal "Conversation"
Advanced pair scribbling. Create a design in 5 minutes. Draw shapes, lines, colors and symbols without talking. This may help reveal how communication works within a family. Parallels may be discovered between the ways clients behave in this situation and the way they behave at home.

Something to Do Together
Promotes sharing of ideas and negotiation. Decide on something you and your art partner would like to do together — like taking a walk — and depict it, including yourselves in the picture.

Painting Completion
Begin a free drawing and pass it to a partner for additions. Continue to pass it back and forth until the process "feels complete."

Building Together
Build something together without verbal interaction. Recycled materials like cardboard tubes and shapes, bits of fabric and yarn are useful to have for this activity.

Back Drawing
One person's back is the canvas. The creator faces the canvas (the partner's back) and "draws" using his/her finger. The "canvas" then transfers onto paper what s/he perceives as the design. Ask the

creator to keep the drawing very simple and work slowly to help the "canvas" comprehend the image. Reverse roles.

Message Sending

Using images or symbols and color/shapes, send a message about yourself to a partner or a message to everyone in the group. Some other ideas include:

1. Send a message to your partner that expresses a positive quality you have noticed and appreciate about him/her.
2. Create a "wish" for your partner.
3. Share a concern you have for your partner.

III. Expression of Inner Feelings

These activities are done to encourage exploration of feelings and fantasies and to create visual representations of them. Anxiety may increase or decrease as a client's awareness of his/her feelings broadens. The therapist may assist a client by clarifying feelings and helping to identify problem-solving strategies.

Behavioral Goals:

Participants will:

*   Express and face their feelings at least once during the session by painting or drawing lines, symbols or forms that represent at least one aspect of how they feel.
*   Express one feeling or mood using at least one color other than black or white.
*   Express at least once nonverbally (through art) to the group something related to a personal problem.
*   Verbally interpret one of his/her drawings to one other person.
*   Interact with one other person by expressing one idea that comes to mind when viewing another person's drawing.
*   Share interest in the feelings of at least two other people by asking at least one question of each about his/her creation.

Affective Words #1
Divide the paper into 6-8 sections. The participants are given about a minute to respond spontaneously with images, color or symbols to key words spoken by the therapist. The words may come from the therapist or be compiled through group brainstorming. Suggestions include words like: love, hate, freedom, responsibility, anger, anxiety, faith, father/mother, trust, rejection, hope, etc. Interesting to use polarities such as: strength/weakness, independence/interdependence. Compare similarities and differences in responses within the group.

Affective Words #2
Write words connoting feelings on small pieces of paper, fold them and place them in a box for the whole group. Shake the box and have each member of the group draw out a piece of paper. Draw or paint what the chosen word means to you without verbalizing the word to the others in the group. Through discussion, the group attempts to match the words with the pictures. Match the correct words with the pictures. Share feelings about the experience.

How Do I Feel Now?
Participants are asked to fold a paper into three sections. In the first section, the client is asked to depict through drawing how s/he is feeling at this moment. In the third section the client responds to the question, "How would you like to feel?" In the middle section, the client tries to express what is in between or what are the steps to feeling better.

Create a Care Package for Yourself
Include both tangible (e.g., cookies, music) and intangible objects (e.g., love, trust, hope) that fit your tastes and needs.

Three Wishes #1
Depict three wishes expressing what you want most out of life. Discussion may then focus on commonalties and differences in the group and also on issues of attainability.

Road of Life (Picture Autobiography) #1
Each participant is asked to depict the road or path of life that s/he has been traveling the past few years (or may go back further). The therapist may suggest the inclusion of three "accomplishments."

Road of Life (Picture Autobiography) #2
Each participant is asked to paint the road or path that s/he has been traveling in life. Then each participant tries to remember how s/he was feeling at certain points along this road. An extension of this work would be depicting in drawing or painting the road a participant hopes to or expects to travel in the future.

Your Future
Participants are asked to divide the paper into three sections. The therapist first asks, "Where will you be in _____ (months? years?)" and then "What will you be doing?" Finally the therapist says, "Look forward five years into the future and portray what you'd like to be doing/who you'd like to be with." Another possible question is: "If you could do anything you really wanted to, what would it be?" These are not easy questions for anyone — try it yourself before you introduce the idea so you can see that it is challenging to predict your future.

Want to Do
Using symbols, images and color, draw a picture of yourself doing something you have never done but always wanted to do. Include in the picture how you think you would feel doing this activity.

Create a Me Collage or Me Box
This project is a kind of autobiography and helps the individual become aware of him/herself in deeper ways. Paint or cover the outside of a box (a small or large box as space allows). Through words, pictures, drawings, stories and photographs use the box to tell about yourself: friends, likes, dislikes, values, plans, experiences, mistakes, etc. The leader can brainstorm categories with the group.

Joy/Sadness/World
Divide the paper into three sections. Think of what it is about the world that brings you joy. It could be the thought that "eagles are no longer endangered" or it could be "nature" in general. Think about your sadness for the world (e.g., hunger, poverty). What do you wish for the world?

Anti-Coloring Book
The anti-coloring book was developed as a creative alternative to the traditional coloring book — which may stifle creativity by giving little room for individual input. There are many books in this series. Each page presents an open-ended question or theme along with the beginning of a drawing to get an individual started. S/he has a lot of leeway to complete the drawing in his/her own way. Some examples of open-ended suggestions that fit the "Expression of Inner Feelings" category are: Do you see your future in the crystal ball? If you went away for a long time, whose portrait would you take with you? What was the nicest dream you ever had? Your worst nightmare?

Events and Emotion
Using the media of your choice, symbolize some of the events and significant, related emotions you have experienced this week.

Association Drawing
An object, event or feeling which is related to a topic (e.g., alcoholism) is drawn by the leader. The drawing is passed around the group for additions from each member that further explain, personalize or communicate a specific meaning.

IV. Self-Perception — Portrayal of Self

To integrate body image with a wider sense of being (e.g., needs, dreams, fears, strengths, values, beliefs).

Behaviors Goals:
Participants will:
- Become more aware of body images or self-concept by drawing themselves and other human figures.
- Interact with others by verbally interpreting their drawings of a person to one or more persons in the art group.
- Become aware of ideas and meanings that can be expressed in symbols in art and demonstrate their understanding of this by using an animal form to express things about themselves.

Hero/Heroine
This is a good activity for identifying qualities that the individual admires and would like to acquire/strengthen in self. Draw the "best" man or woman you could be or your hero/heroine. When the drawing is complete, turn the paper over and write a few sentences explaining what it is about this individual you admire. Can you see these qualities in yourself or the potential for developing these qualities or attributes in some degree?

Immediate States of Being
Select one of the following phrases to paint or draw: "I am," "I feel," "I have" or "I do." On completion, exchange and discuss paintings or drawings with a partner. Then select a second phrase and do another painting/drawing. Exchange and discuss with a different partner. Exchange impressions about each other's feelings.

Self Book
If you wrote a book about yourself, what would it be titled? Draw the cover and write the forward.

Self Portrait on Paper
This can be an evocative activity and most likely would be done with a group that has developed some trust in the leader and other members. On one sheet of paper, using any media, depict yourself as you would really like to be (ideal self). On another piece of pa-

per, depict yourself as you believe you really are (perceived/real self). Discussion could include questions like: What is different about these two images? What steps/behavior/changes could reduce the gap between these two images?

Animal Side
Choose one or both exercises:
- Depict yourself as the kind of animal(s) you feel you are most like.
- Depict yourself as the animal you would least like to be.

Discuss or write about your feelings about your choice(s).

Inside/Outside Box
This activity is a variation on the "Me Box" concept. Use a box to depict two aspects of self. On the outside depict the parts of yourself that you think others see. On the inside of the box show your inside self and your personal qualities. Write about or discuss your feelings about any differences that may appear.

Body Tracing
This activity requires a lot of floor space. Using a sheet of butcher paper the length of your body, have someone trace your outline as you lie on the paper. Generally people stretch out full length on the paper but you could assume a position (e.g., fetal) that had some meaning for you. Embellish the inside with colors, symbols and images that tell about you, your feelings, your state of health.

Self Poster
Using any media, make a poster of yourself that addresses the following questions:
1. How does your body feel?
2. Think of healing. What images come to mind?
3. Include what is important to you in your life.

Masks
Mask and mask making falls under the category of "Portrayal of Self" and is dealt with extensively in the *Masks* chapter.

Morning Mirror
Draw or paint: What do you look like when you first get up in the morning?

Positive/Negative Attributes
• Draw/paint three positive characteristics of self.
• Draw/paint one negative characteristic/aspect of self.
Discuss individuals' depictions — how realistic are they? — in the group.
Variations: Express two positive aspects about yourself, pass papers around in order for other participants to add qualities.
Divide a piece of paper in half. Depict feelings you would like to get rid of and attributes you would like to develop.

What I Like About Myself
Have each participant create his/her own territory in the room using a piece of butcher paper, making sure his/her name is located visibly on the paper. Through the use of words, abstract symbols, pictures from magazines and images, depict your positive qualities — the things about yourself you like (may be qualities, interests, accomplishments). Participants then move around the room and add on to one another's butcher paper territories the additional qualities they feel you have. "Post-its" notes work great for this purpose. At the end of the activity, discuss what the individual initially did and what was added on and by whom.

Heroic Deed
Draw, paint and write: You have just performed a heroic deed. This is the picture and the story in the newspaper the next day.

Award
Draw or paint: Award yourself a medal for what you know you do best.

Johari Window Exercise
Depict the proportions that fit for you in various situations and discuss how you might change those proportions. (See Chapter 4, *Groups*, for a complete discussion of Johari Windows and how to determine the proportions for each block.)

Status Change
Through a photo or drawing collage, depict your daily life, ____ years ago (your choice) and your daily life now. Write about or discuss your feelings about each situation.

Positive Lifetime Review
Note: This technique will take several sessions to complete. Create an album which will show positive aspects of your life experience. These may include incidents from your past, childhood memories, school activities, family happenings, work experiences, situations which offered pleasure, vacations, friends, social affiliations, hobbies or sports activities. Any recall which has a positive association can be shown through a representational or abstract portrayal. Memories put into a concrete form may give an individual the opportunity to see the wealth of experience s/he has accrued. May strengthen self-identification, increase self-esteem and/or stimulate further recall.

Life Line Drawing
Draw a picture that traces your life from your birth until sometime in the future. Mark the important events in your life along the line in some way. This can be with pictures, designs or whatever images/symbols you like. You can use crayons, markers, pencils or whatever is available. It can be as large or as small as you like.

Personal Shield

This shield represents some important parts of you and shows what your goals are. Complete the four sections of the shield:
1. Three photos or pictures that describe me.
2. (Draw or write) Three things that I'm good at.
3. (Draw or write) A present I would give to myself.
4. My favorite animal or an animal that is like me.

Colors, size or shape of any pictures s/he would like to draw are up to the individual.

I Am a Tree

Draw yourself as a tree — thinking about the kind of tree that most represents who you are. Taking turns, each individual holds up his/her completed drawing and describes the tree, speaking in the first person about the characteristics of the tree. Example: I am strong, I have lots of energy; or I am frail and delicate, I am standing in a storm. Will my roots hold me? Then have each member pass their drawing to the person on the right, so that everyone has someone else's drawing. Repeat the descriptive process with this new drawing, again taking on the characteristics that you see in the drawing, speaking in the first person. Each person will see new adjectives for the drawings and will be expressing a new part of themselves. For example, a strong individual might be exploring a part of themselves by expressing the statement, "I am delicate." Descriptions should be kept to a couple of minutes at the most; one or two adjectives are fine. Repeat the process as often as time allows, hopefully until the drawings return to the original owner. You could divide the group to facilitate the process. Follow with a discussion of feelings that emerged.

Variations:
1. Depict yourself as a house and describe your characteristics (e.g., size, color, style, outside, inside). What kinds of furniture or objects are there? What does the house feel like when you walk inside?

2. Portray yourself as a symbol. Examples: a thunderbolt, a cloud, a heart. Verbally give some clues about yourself without showing the picture. Example: thunderbolt, "I make a lot of sudden noise that unsettles people." The participants will try to guess the aspect of self you are portraying.

Influences
Depict three things that have influenced your life greatly, including people, places, ideas, beliefs and experiences.

V. Interpersonal Relations
To make participants more aware of others and the way others perceive them.

Behavioral Goals:
*   Become more aware of the interactions between people.
*   Increase understanding of family dynamics as they relate to the current situation.
*   Learn to see oneself from other people's points of view.

Support
Depict a time in your life when you needed support and in what form(s) that support came to you. Example: loss of a family member. The support came from church members who called and sent cards and from grieving sessions with a therapist.

Portraits
In pairs, group members draw one another adding qualities, characteristics and aspects to create the most complete representation of the person.

Care Packages for Others
Create care packages for one another. Include both tangible (e.g., chocolate, furry slippers) and intangible gifts (e.g., love, trust, hope) that fit that individual's personality and needs.

Your Family
Using drawing, collage, photographs or clay, depict your family.

Family Sociogram
Create a sociogram model of your family. A sociogram is a visual diagram showing the members of a group and how they relate to/feel about each other. You may use circles of colored paper to represent various individuals.

Kinetic Family
Depict the family doing something together or a typical family scene.

Animal Family
Depict family members as animals that most represent their personalities and/or behavior.

Mural
Mural making can be an enjoyable and also revealing activity. You can learn:
- how people cooperate (e.g., deciding who uses what space and how much space)
- how boundaries are created (e.g., invasion of "your" space by another member).
- different styles in approaching the project (e.g., thoughtful, slow or impulsive, quick).

Taking a piece of butcher paper long enough to enable everyone to contribute to the project, create a mural on topics, including:
1. Group mural. Portray your "ward," community, class or group. Note positive and negative aspects of the group.
2. Nature collage. Depict nature in a way that says something about you. Example: the ocean environment can be stormy or calm, it has riches hidden under the surface.

3. Global issues. Have your mural say something about world is-
    sues that concern you (e.g., violence, peace).

Group Mobile
Each person adds something that expresses an aspect of
him/herself. Example: a pair of sunglasses (I am hiding my expressions), a transparent cloth (you all can see through me).

Unfinished Messages
Use the collage method to depict family, friends or acquaintances
with whom you left something unsaid. Write or tell what you wish
you were able to say to each of these people.

I Give You
Complete the statement, "I give you the gift of _____" using any
medium to express a characteristic or quality.

Circle of Love
Place yourself in the center of a piece of paper. Depict the circle of
love that surrounds you — your family (alive or deceased), friends,
animals or energies from nature or places (e.g., home).

Trophy
To whom would you give a trophy and what would it look like?

Family Crest
Design a family crest that tells something about you and your family.

Birthday
Draw or use other media and answer the question: Today is your
birthday. Can you see the gift you want most in the world?

As Seen by Others
Each person receives an 11" x 14" sheet of paper on which they
write their name. Arrange the seating into a circle and ask every-

one to pass their sheet of paper to the person on the right. Each person is to cut something (a word or picture) out of a magazine which reminds them of something they like about the person whose sheet they have. They then paste it on and pass the sheet to the right. Once everyone receives his/her own sheet, they look it over for a minute. Next each person holds up his/her collage while other members describe why they chose to paste on what they did.

VI. The Individual's Place in His/Her World

To increase awareness of each of our relationships to the world.

Behavioral Goals:
- Learning to share space with other people.
- Seeing one's place as part of the whole world.

Sharing Space with Another
Sit facing a partner and draw together on one piece of paper without speaking. Be aware of territoriality and how it is affected by your particular relationship with another person.

House, Tree, Person
Include all three in a picture.

Elements
Respond to the elements of fire, water, earth and air in a drawing or painting.

Your World
Using the concept of the sociogram, design your world. Include the people that you feel close to, places that have meaning, your interests, values or dreams.

Time Tree

Depict yourself as a tree in three stages of growth — yesterday, today and tomorrow. After you have drawn these three images, answer the following questions:

- Where are you growing?
- What are your strengths? Weaknesses?
- What nurtures you?
- What is your future?
- What might you change?

Create the World

As a group, create an image of the world. Any of the following themes could be used:

- Identify wishes for the world's healing.
- Share sadness for the world.
- Create your ideal world.
- Depict what brings you joy in the world and what brings you sadness.

This activity, with its various parts, could be effective as a mural process.

Then and Now

Depict the world, or your world, as it was and then as it is.

7

Masks

Masks...we all wear them. They can be helpful or destructive, self-made or imposed upon us. They are denied and confessed; they can be used to reveal or to conceal. They can be cemented, nailed, glued or hinged. They may be taped or painted directly onto one's face. Behind each one may lie recognized feelings and unfamiliar ones...feelings that may have been suppressed, distorted or protected.

The power of masks as a therapeutic tool, therefore, is enormous. They possess a tremendous potential for facilitating growth, understanding and even, in the course of this, enjoyment. They also may serve as a powerful reminder of what we already know.

This discussion of masks is a segue between art and drama, at least historically, because drama (as well as dance) once naturally proceeded from the art of mask making. Masks are an ancient form of expression used to celebrate earth forces and cycles; to communicate with the spiritual realm; to thrust the wearer into a different persona and set of behaviors. By putting on a mask, the wearer suspends everyday reality and can dance, act or sing about experiences outside of the tangible. Masks have been used across the ages and around the world.

Mask Creation in a Therapeutic Context

- Participants may want to decorate one or two sides of a mask — they may even choose to do several. Many aspects of the self (internal vs. external, different personalities, ideal self) can be depicted in this way.
- Always allow for self-description or self-disclosure.
- Showing examples can sometimes encourage or spark creativity as long as no comparisons are made.
- The leader is most effective when creating his/her own mask, too. (Be conscious of what you are disclosing to the group.)
- Once made, masks can be worn, interpreted, traded and passed around. Other group members can contribute to understanding by expressing what they think a person is saying or trying to say, or by pointing out a person's patterns of expression.

Masks as Therapy

The following section groups suggestions for creating and using certain types of masks according to five different therapeutic issues (self-esteem, physical or body awareness, imagination/creativity, social skills and rapport building).

As every therapy group is different, these can only be suggestions — there are a wide range of issues which can be explored using this medium. Within each category, any activity will be more or less appropriate to do with any of the masks created. They are meant to be "mixed and matched." These activities may be even further interchanged, and new ones added, as a therapist recognizes other applications and contexts for them. Read about theater games (Chapter 9) and refer back to masks to see if any of the ideas from that section can be applied. If and when possible, have the participants wear their masks during the activity. As stated previously, the mask is a vehicle for entering another reality and can enable the wearer to gain greater insight into the self.

Self-Esteem

The mask depicts:

How others see you or how you would like to be seen by a friend

The person you would like to become

Combine the above suggestions and create a mask with two sides

Your uniqueness/your strengths

When you have felt your best

What you like/dislike about yourself

How you feel when you are frightened, happy, etc.

An image from a dream

Yourself as a child, adolescent or adult

Yourself as a child, adult or parent (transactional analysis model)

Use masks to:

Introduce yourself in the present: "I am _____," and name the areas of yourself that you want to strengthen (e.g., trust).

Introduce yourself the way your best friend, family member or other significant person in your life would.

Answer this Orff Schulwerk rondo (see Chapter 12 for details of this technique):
Masks can be happy, masks can be sad,
What about your mask makes you glad?

Fantasize that you just went to the "Magic Shop" and got more of some personal quality that you want. Introduce yourself and describe how that quality helps you in your life.

Project the future: role play meeting a friend/another patient from your treatment program in 1 year/5 years. Talk about your lives.

Create a "Symphony of Emotions" Theater Game. Each participant produces a sound which relates the emotion that is portrayed on his/her mask. The leader "orchestrates" these sounds, by cueing the participants to start or stop, and lower or raise the volume or pace.

Have a conversation with your mask: give each "sub-personality" a name and a statement that would typical for that part of yourself. You may ask other members of the group to portray each sub-personality.

Physical or Body Awareness

Masks tend to be limited to the face and exclude the rest of the body. Full body tracing or tracings of specific body parts invite a fuller understanding and a more holistic exploration of feelings.

The mask depicts:	Activities:
How a little creature living inside you might see you	Interpret your mask through movement and/or sounds.
Yourself as a: flower, sky, tree, stream	If possible, tape or safety pin the body mask to your back so that it moves as you move. In motion it "relates" to others and takes on a life of its own
Your favorite/least favorite parts	

Imagination and Creativity

We can be or feel whatever we want to — there is no limit to our imaginations. By encouraging participants to project themselves into new worlds and experiences they may be able to get in touch with and experience who or what they would like to be. This is the time to bring out the props, the hats, magic wands and crystal balls — whatever helps to create the illusion and enhance the fantasy.

The mask depicts:

Your favorite fantasy, comic or storybook character

What you would like to be like when you grow up/mature/in 5 years/in 10 years…

Yourself in a another age, past or future

Yourself in heaven

Yourself after your death

Yourself as the happiest/most evil/wisest person in the world

Activities:

Be your hero/heroine. Identify qualities or behaviors you respect in them. Let this come through your actions in handling what you or the leader would consider difficult role play situations.

Make up a story about the mask you made.

Use various masks (with two or three person groups) to create and stage a story or scene.

Play "Roving Reporter." Each group member becomes a character who moves, thinks and speaks in a unique way. (See the "Radio and TV Exercise" in the *Theater Games* chapter to help direct the group in this.)

Suggestions are taken for setting — a school, an African plain, etc. The roving reporter (often the leader at first), circulates through the room, interviewing characters. Characters mill around until commanded to "freeze." The reporter picks a character and interviews him/her while the others listen.

Social Skills

Social skills improve when we learn to understand the world from another person's point of view. These masks let us take on the role of another person so we can learn his/her way of dealing with situations. Masks are also useful in letting us practice using a characteristic such as assertiveness that might be too difficult to use in our normal way of being.

The mask or hat depicts:

People who experience varying degrees of comfort in social situations. A person's behavior might be: talkative, shy, rude, vulnerable, happy, competitive, snobbish

People of different cultures, races or abilities/disabilities

People in positions of authority, such as teachers, doctors or police officers

Activities:

Create role play situations for one another. Choose situations that would challenge and/or strengthen some quality in each person's character. The shy person may be challenged to stand up to a police officer's questions, for example. Choose real life situations.

Create 2 or 3 character situations in which to practice the following behaviors:
- Giving appropriate greetings
- Saying "no!"
- Beginning a conversation
- Sharing appreciation

"Try on" the experience of being someone with his/her individual perspective and problems. This may help to bridge cultural and personal differences and promote empathy, respect and/or insight into others. Group makes suggestions for role play situations.

Rapport Building

Rapport building is important in making a group come together. These activities are designed to be done as a group project to allow the members of the group to get to know one another better.

Make masks in a group:

Create life masks

Each person in a small group (3-4 members) begins working on his/her own mask. After a certain period of time, each person passes his/her mask to the person on the right. This continues until everyone receives his/her mask back.

In small groups (3-4 people) each participant makes masks of the other group members.

Group activities:

Create a mask mural.

Exchange masks with a partner. Look at the mask, wear it, experience what it feels like to have it on. Make a few statements that seem to fit and make up a movement to go with the mask. Return it to the owner. Discuss what happened.

Mingle around the room, talking with different people about the process of creating your mask and what it represents.

Pass each mask around the group. Each person may tell the group one thought about the mask.

Place all masks in the middle of the floor. Each person chooses one and takes on the character of that mask, gives his/her interpretation of the mask or creates an experience from the mask.

Body Sculpting: One person wears a mask while his/her partner(s) sculpt or move him/her as a puppet. Remind the "clay" or "puppet" to relax and let the partner(s) move him/her.

Processes of Mask Creation

Many materials are appropriate for mask making. Visit a natural history museum to get an inkling of the possibilities for creating masks. Some of the materials that the group leader might want to have available for construction include:

- paper — all sorts, including construction and crepe paper
- craft materials — corrugated cardboard, cardboard tubes, fabrics, yarn
- decorative materials — sequins, beads, feathers, etc.
- art supplies — markers, paints, crayons, oil pastels
- ceramic supplies — if you have access to a kiln, wonderful masks can be shaped out of clay, fired and glazed
- papier maché materials (see process below)
- plaster gauze (see process below)
- face paints — an easy way to create masks, especially fun for children.

For better results and easier clean-up, use a good, water-based product like Aquarelle Caran D'Ache which is applied with a brush.

Papier Maché

These masks are inexpensive and fairly easy to make. If the budget allows and/or the group is small, it is now possible to purchase paper pulp that mixes with water. A mask can then be formed by spreading this mixture over a blown-up balloon. This is a fast and easy medium for mask making. If the group is large or resources are limited, use the traditional newspaper and glue method, also known as papier maché.

Materials: newspaper and newspaper strips, masking tape, wheat paste (for wallpapering) or common starch (watered down slightly), good latex balloons (flimsier balloons may burst while the mask is being worked on), paints (acrylics are preferable), gesso (optional), clear spray glossy finish (optional, unless the there is a concern that the paints being used might flake or peel over time).

1. Inflate a latex balloon to medium size. Don't overfill. Overfilling may cause the balloon to burst as the newspaper strips are laid down or may create too much surface area to work on.
2. Roll up a newspaper into the shape of a horseshoe. This will act as a cradle for the balloon. Tape this to the table and then tape the balloon gently to the horseshoe.
3. Cut or rip newspaper into 2" x 4-6" strips. Some strips will need to be shorter to fit contours like the nose area.
4. Make up liquid mixture. Follow directions on the package for wheat paste. Remember to ask if anyone has wheat allergies and to use rubber gloves to prevent the development of a rash. If using starch, add a little water to thin it for easy use. Make sure there is good ventilation because the starch can have a strong smell.
5. Dip the strip of newspaper into the mixture and remove the excess. Work from top to bottom, crisscrossing layers for extra strength.
6. To build a nose or planes of face or forehead, roll newspaper pieces or paper towel pieces and tape them down with masking tape. This makes the temporary structure to place strips on until enough have been laid down to hold additional strips in place. Tissue paper can also be used for an interesting surface texture over layers of newspaper.
7. Build a total of 4 or 5 layers (about 1/8-1/4" thick) for strength.
8. Leave the mask undisturbed for several days until thoroughly dry and no longer cool to the touch.
9. Apply gesso, if desired. Gesso is a primer that covers the newspaper and creates a base for the paint. One advantage to using gesso is that less paint will be required to cover a mask.
10. Paint in desired colors. Make sure to wait for one coat to dry before painting over any spot with another color (e.g., painting eyes over the face color). Be patient — the results will be worth the wait. A heat tool or hair dryer can speed up the drying process.

11. When thoroughly dry, spray with acrylic gloss finish for durability and water resistance.
12. Finally, glue on any decorative items such as feathers, sequins or beads.

Making a Life Mask Using Plaster Gauze

Those of us who are lucky enough to be or know a theater student, or to have contact with someone involved in doing special effects for movies, may have had the opportunity to have a life mask made of their face in latex. It is an interesting experience, but not one for the claustrophobic. The whole idea of making life masks can be frightening for some people, not just for those suffering from claustrophobia, but also for individuals who have difficulty with touching or trust. By using plaster gauze, the potential for claustrophobic feelings can be dealt with by limiting the amount of surface covered by the plaster. Resolving touch or trust issues is more difficult — partners should be directed to be thoughtful and gentle in both touch and voice, and to stop if the process becomes uncomfortable for either of them.

Materials: Plaster gauze (a material formerly used in making casts; made by Johnson and Johnson, it is also available in good craft stores), old clothes, shower caps or hair pins to protect hair, towels or newspaper, bowls with water, scissors, Vaseline, baby powder.

1. Make sure to wear old clothes.
2. Pair up with another person and take turns making the masks.
3. The person having the mask made should thoroughly cover his/her face (including any facial hair or hair lying close to the face) with Vaseline. This averts undesirable consequences such as pulling off eyebrow hairs as the mask is pulled off! Also pin back hair or use a shower cap to cover it.

4. The person then lies on a towel or a layer of newspapers. This makes the work easier for the partner but isn't strictly necessary. The person can sit in a chair or wheelchair if necessary.

5. The "sculptor" has cut a gauze roll into 2" by 3-4" strips and set them aside. S/he begins by dipping the strips into the water and removing the excess. Don't leave the strips in the water as this will remove all the plaster. Beginning from top to bottom, cover one entire area before moving to a new area. Crisscross for strength. Covering the eyes or mouth with plaster is *not* recommended. In order to cover the mouth, for example, it would be necessary to insert straws in the nose to facilitate breathing. This is not a pleasant or desirable experience.

6. Create a surface that is about 1/8-1/4" thick. The layers underneath will start to harden first. Feel with a finger to determine whether an area needs strengthening with more strips. Make any additions to the mask immediately after removing it and while it is still drying.

7. Let it dry once all the layers are applied. After about 5 minutes, ask the person under the mask to make some facial motions. If the mask begins to move away easily from the face it is time to gently remove the mask. Once removed, it is possible to remove the sticky feel of the Vaseline from inside the mask by sprinkling baby powder onto the inner surface.

8. Some professionals like to blend the texture of the gauze by working a bit of plaster into the mask surface. Use some of the plaster that has fallen off the gauze for this purpose.

9. Paint and spray with acrylic gloss finish for protection.

10. Decorate with other items if desired.

8

An Introduction to Drama Therapy Groups

Many excellent therapeutic techniques have their origin in the theater. From theater games to psychodrama, these involve clients in a world of imagination and possibility which has relevance to behaviors (their own and other's) in the larger world beyond the stage.

Although the goals of the various drama therapies may be different, many of the techniques and processes of the drama group are the same across the board. The following is a broad outline for conducting drama therapy in a group.

Levels of Therapies

- **Theater Games.** These are used to increase spontaneity and interaction within a group, and often form the basis for other group work.
- **Role Playing.** Used to work on changing behaviors or introducing new ones. A problem solving technique.

- **Sociodrama.** Used in a group which is working on common problems, to help the group gain insights into behaviors that they all share.
- **Psychodrama.** Centers on one person's problems and aims to help that person reach a deeper understanding of his/her behavior and/or a resolution of emotional conflicts.

Common Objectives

Not all of these objectives are shared by every type of drama therapy, but there is considerable overlap. The objectives are to:

- Increase interaction: this is often done through the use of theater games and improvisation to increase and develop trust. The emphasis is on group trust and group interaction.
- Release and control emotions: again, often accomplished through the use of theater games. The leader functions as director, steering the course of the dramatic action.
- Break behavioral and role patterns which are not constructive.
- Gain insight into familiar patterns.
- Gain insight into alternative patterns.
- Explore conflicts and different responses to them.
- Increase spontaneity.
- Increase self-esteem and self-confidence.
- Provide a learning situation that is fun and reinforcing of positive behaviors.

Process

- Group warm-ups
- Pair warm-ups
- Improvisational scene/Role play/Dramatic scene
- Declimaxing — Closure for entire group

General Guidelines

- Approach and begin at the level where clients "are at." Don't force a greater intensity of dramatic action than they are ready to handle.
- Resistance and passivity are often seen in clients at the beginning of a session, and need to be addressed and worked through.
- Create structure. It increases the feelings of safety in the group.
- Remember the element of "surprise" to increase spontaneity.
- Exaggerating behavior (yours, or a reflection of a group member's) can instill humor in a situation, *if* there is enough trust.
- Make sure each session is designed to promote success.

Warm-Up Exercises

The following exercises can be used with any drama group.

Essences

This activity can be done in verbal or written form. If done verbally, participants form a circle. Each participant has a chance to answer one of the following questions. Several questions may be asked in sequence. If the answers are written, each participant has a chance to read what s/he has written, or answers may be exchanged and discussed in pairs.

- If you could go anywhere in the world, where would you go?
- If you could be anyone (living or deceased), who would you be?
- If you won the lottery, what would you do? How would your life change?
- If you could invent something, what would it be?
- If you could live at any time in the past, present or future, which would you choose?
- If you could discover something, what would it be?
- If you could win an award, what would it be for?

Personal
- If you could change your name, would you?
- If you could make a wish for yourself, what would it be?
- If you could receive the perfect present, what would it be?
- Plan your perfect day.
- Is there something you would like to hear from someone (friend, relative)?
- Introduce yourself the way your best friend would.

Projective: *Who we are/How we see others*
Use questions such as these to ask about a person in the group. Describing yourself as a kind off thing can be a lot less threatening than describing yourself as a kind of person.
- If you were a _____, what kind would you be?
- If _____ were a _____, what kind would s/he be?

Fill in the blanks with some of these objects.

• flower	• season	• transportation
• color	• food	• perfume
• movement	• jewel	• book
• piece of furniture	• holiday	• landscape
• sound	• song	• sport
• weather	• smell	• musical instrument
• ice cream	• animal	
• fabric	• movie	

Interpersonal Exercises
- Empty chair technique (details in the Psychodrama section of Chapter 10, *Drama*).
- Appreciations/Resentments: expressed to group members.
- Is there something you would like to hear from someone in this group?
- Send a message to everyone in the group.

Suggestions for Agreements in the Group

To create an environment that is "safe" for emotional release and discovery, it is important to set up agreements with members of the group.

- Only one person talks at a time. Be respectful of others.
- Talk to someone, not about him/her. Don't treat someone as if s/he isn't present.
- Each person's pace is respected. We all open up, grow, release at different rates.
- No one is forced to participate. The goal is to reinforce individual responsibility for participation, so that it can be carried over into other life situations.
- It is not acceptable to disrupt the group.
- Do not analyze.
- In sharing and giving feedback, respond subjectively (e.g., How has the drama touched you? What have you experienced that related to ___'s experience?)

9

Theater Games and Improvisation

All the world's a stage,
and all the men and women in it merely players...
... And one man in his time plays many parts,
His acts being seven ages...

— William Shakespeare

Shakespeare may have said it best: we are part of an ever unfolding drama, life, that casts us in a variety of roles and situations. We begin as small babies, charming our families. As children we cast ourselves as heroes, princesses and princes, animals and characters out of our favorite books, TV shows, and movies. In adolescence and adulthood, we take on the roles of lovers, parents, workers and friends, while middle age and retirement present us with new roles: mentoring, grandparenting and retirement. Along the way we each develop our own script and a set of behaviors to help us play it. One of the goals of theater games is to help clients to become aware of, and perhaps reflect on, the many roles they've played in their own lives. Most people would not classify themselves as actors in the sense of Hollywood or Broadway stars, but need to be reminded that they have acted out challenging situations and a variety of personalities. Players in theater draw from their experiences in life and they can, too.

"Improvisation" is the term for creating theater in the moment, drawing only on the techniques or resources at hand and without any preparation. It is "working without a net." Theater games are the tools of improvisation, used for sharpening the skills of the players and for creating theater.

Theater Games are exercises or techniques that have at their root the following beliefs and attributes:

- **Allow experimentation.** There is no "right" or "wrong" way to improvise.
- **Encourage spontaneity.** Theater games are first and foremost "artifices" against artificiality — structures designed to almost "fool" spontaneity into being. Through spontaneity we are "re-formed" into ourselves, we (re)discover our truer selves and a more authentic way of behaving. Spontaneity, the core element of theater games, is the moment of personal freedom when we are faced with a reality, see it, explore it and act accordingly.
- **Involve problem solving and creative challenges.** For example, if a player is asked to become one of the cogs in an imaginary machine, s/he must first identify how s/he will sound and move and then how to fit with the other human parts of the machine.
- **Focus concentration.** A key element of drama — it enables the player to be present, open, ready to react to and participate in the exploration and resolution of a situation.
- **Encourage intuitive responses.** These can only be made in "the here and now," the immediate moment. A player learns to react to what is happening in the moment. It is almost impossible to "plan ahead" if there is no script and no way to know ahead of time how others will behave. This experience develops trust in self and affects overall self-esteem.

- **People learn through experience and experiencing.** No one teaches anyone anything.
- **Increase openness.** If the environment permits it, anyone can learn whatever s/he chooses to learn. If the individual permits it, the environment will teach him/her everything it has to teach.
- **"Talent" is not required.** Anyone can participate. "Talented behavior," according to Viola Spolin (1983) who is the originator of theater games, "may be simply a greater individual capacity for experiencing...It is in the increasing of the individual capacity for experiencing that the untold potentiality of a personality can be evoked."

Aspects of Spontaneity

In **Improvisation for the Theater**, Viola Spolin (1983) outlines seven aspects of spontaneity (elements which are connected to its development or its impact on behavior):

1. **Games.** Games provide a form for inviting involvement and for encouraging the personal freedom necessary for genuine experiencing. Through engaging in play, a person is learning skills, having fun, relating to others and feeling the freedom that makes one open to experiences. Ingenuity and inventiveness are encouraged and applauded. The person can reach the objective of the game in any manner or style s/he chooses, as long as s/he abides by the rules (freedom within structure). Any game worth playing is highly social and has a problem that needs solving within it. Learning is the result of solving the problem in an effective way.

2. **Approval/disapproval.** The first step toward being able to play is feeling personal freedom and understanding that there is no right or wrong way to solve a problem. Looking for approval or disapproval in others is creatively paralyzing. With an emerging sense of self, the need for authoritarianism drops

away, and intuitive awareness emerges. Working through problems that arise, in subject matter or interpretation, allows them to be seen not as problems but as a means of increasing the knowledge of everyone in the group, including the facilitator.

3.   **Group expression.** This is truly an art form in which the "sum of the parts is greater than the whole." Each person's energy, enthusiasm and ideas are important to the success of the group improvisation. At the same time, each member must be a part of the group relationship. Through awareness exercises and heightened sensory receptors the members become each other's arms, legs and actions. Competition is not helpful; cooperation is. The goal of these exercises is for players to be able to work interdependently with full individual participation.

4.   **Audience.** An audience is what makes performance meaningful. In improvisation the audience participates in the unfolding of theater. The player becomes freer with the understanding that the audience comes not to judge or encourage but, as a group, is there to share an experience with the actors. The actors and the audience are actually partners in creation.

5.   **Theater techniques.** These are techniques of communicating. Achieving communication is more important than the methods used. Whatever the techniques, they are just tools to help sharpen awareness, thinking and relating skills so that the individuals can respond to a variety of new situations and experiences.

6.   **Carrying the learning process into daily life.** There are no lines to learn, no characters to research in improvisation. Through sharpening one's sensory equipment the player can make direct, fresh contact with the environment, people and objects in his/her world. The individual who develops a wider view of the world is richer in all aspects of life.

7.   **Physicalization.** This term describes the means by which material is presented to the player on a physical, non-verbal level as opposed to an intellectual or psychological approach. The experience is concrete and immediate. An important goal of

theater games is to encourage freedom of physical expression, which opens the door for insight. The player experiences a more direct perception of the world — and a more open self in relation to it.

Viola Spolin's Theater Games

When facilitating/directing theater games it is helpful to have space set up that invites participation. Players should be arranged so that they can be ready to join in at any time. This is accomplished by having everyone sit or stand in a semi-circle facing a center that is designated as "on-stage." The facilitator/director takes part in the group.

Orientation Game
Description: Orientation is an important step in introducing improvisation to new players. It is the first step in learning to create reality (e.g., objects, feelings, situations) for the player and others.
Directions: One player goes on-stage, picks a simple activity and begins doing it (e.g., painting a fence, raking leaves, cooking, sweeping the floor) without verbal or sound cues. Others come on stage one at a time and join in doing this activity. Players can join in even if they don't know initially what is going on. This is a good starting point for physicalization.

The activity may also be done in partners. When rapport has been established in the group, it's a great learning experience for one member (who has an idea) to take another member (who has no idea what is going on) to center stage and begin an activity. For example, the initiating player might begin the movement of combing and cutting hair. When the other player realizes what is being portrayed, s/he joins in and responds by being the client. Players are amazed to find that they can be engaged in an activity before they even know exactly what they are doing.

Variation: Players do an activity in pairs while other members guess the activity. Examples: tennis, volleyball, checkers, doing nails, cooking, hanging pictures or watching TV, movies or sports.

Observation Game
Description: Helps sharpen observation and concentration skills.
Directions: A dozen or more real objects are placed on a tray which is set in the center of the circle of players. After approximately 15 seconds, the tray is covered or removed. The players make individual lists (could also be done in pairs) of as many objects as they can remember. The lists are then compared to the tray of objects.

Involvement in 3's and 4's
Description: Players need to demonstrate cooperation in order to accomplish the task.
Directions: The group is divided into smaller groups of 3 or 4. Each group agrees on an imaginary object which cannot be used without involving all of them. They are to participate in a joint action in which all move the same thing. The group's objective is to make the object seem visible to the audience. Examples of actions: rolling up a fishing net, pushing a stalled car, tugging a boat in/out of the water, taffy pulling.

How Old Am I ?
Description: This exercise gives players an opportunity to explore their conceptions and possible stereotypes of age and allows them to put themselves in another person's place.
Directions: Facilitator/Director sets up a simple "Where," preferably a bus stop. A "bench" (chair, stool, etc.) is set up facing the audience. A player writes down an age on slip of paper and gives it to the director before going on stage. The player acts out this age while being in the established setting. If, for example, a bus stop is used, the player portraying a child might skip on stage chewing gum and then play with a yo-yo, fidget, fumble for change. If the

player is portraying an adult, s/he might walk briskly onstage carrying a briefcase, sit down and make notes, pace and/or often look at a wristwatch. Props may be real or imaginary. The rest of the group guesses the player's age.

The Where Game
Description: Similar to orientation games, this helps focus the player on communicating a physical awareness of *Where* the action is taking place. In *Where* games players learn to work in three environments: the immediate, the general and the larger. The immediate environment is the area closest to us (e.g., the table at which we are eating and all the related objects). The general environment is the room in which the table is placed, with its doors, windows and other aspects. The larger environment is the area beyond the room — outside the window — the birds, trees, landscape.
Directions: A player goes on stage and shows us *Where* through his/her use of objects in the immediate and general environment. When another player thinks s/he knows *Where* the player is, s/he assumes a character (a "*Who*"), enters the *Where* and develops a relationship with the first player. Others join them, one at a time, in a similar fashion. Suggestions for environments include: library, supermarket, airport, hospital, beach, art gallery, restaurant and school.

Weather Exercise
Description: Sharpens the player's awareness of the environment and how it affects his/her body.
Directions: A player goes on stage and shows what kind of weather or climate s/he is experiencing. The other players try to guess the weather conditions — then a new player comes on stage. The group processes the activity asking questions such as: Did the weather envelop him/her? Did the player use his/her body to show us the weather? (e.g., heat — adjusting clothing that is sticking to the body; mopping sweat off face, taking off shoes). Did s/he focus on the weather or on a character? On the weather or a situation?

Word Game
Description: Similar to Charades.
Directions: Divide into teams. Each team selects a word that can be divided into syllables that also form individual words. (Words could be chosen ahead of time by the director and then picked out of a hat to facilitate the process.) For example, the word "industrial" divides into: "inn," "dust," and "trial." The group tries to guess the words being enacted. Other word suggestions: window (win doe), planet (plan eat), carpool (car pool). Actor tries to convey the words to the rest of his/her team without speaking by using pantomime (gestures, movements and facial expressions).
Variation: Use the standard Charades format with each person acting out a phrase such as a movie or song title without speaking.

Body Sculpting in Pairs
Description: Develops sensitivity to another person's character and increases spatial awareness.
Directions: Divide group into pairs. One person in each pair starts out as the sculptor and the other person as the "clay." Take turns as sculptor arranging the partner's body to show his/her personality (or some aspect of it) as you perceive it.

Body Sculpting in Fours
Description: Sharpens clients' sense of touch and space awareness.
Directions: Form groups of four. One person is the sculptor and another person is the clay. The other two people close their eyes. The sculptor sculpts the clay into a statue. The two people with eyes closed then become the new sculptor and the new clay, *Keeping his/her eyes closed,* the new sculptor feels the statue and attempts to reproduce it using the person who has become the second piece of clay. Upon completion compare the sculptures.

Radio and TV Exercise — Roving Reporter

Description: The goals are to exercise the imagination, to think quickly and to have a social experience.

Directions: The director asks for a suggestion of a place or situation (e.g., the Olympic Games, now or early days). The players are instructed to assume a character of any age or background (can be famous or everyday persons) and interact with the immediate environment of that place. The player who acts as the interviewer will freeze the action when an interview is going to take place by saying "freeze." This enables all the players to hear what is said during the interview. The Roving Reporter or interviewer circulates through the crowd until s/he interviews all the players.

Prop Round

Description: A good warm-up activity which also helps develop creative thinking ability.

Direction: Players sit in a circle. A prop is passed around the circle and each player has to transform it from what it was originally intended for into something new and different. For example, an empty toilet paper roll could be a telephone receiver or a bullhorn. An idea for use cannot be repeated. The other players in the circle must guess what the object is before it can be passed on. If a player cannot think of another use, he may simply pass the object on. Continue the activity around the circle until the players are having a difficult time thinking up new ideas.

Paper Bag Dramatics

Description: Exercises creativity and cooperation skills.

Directions: Divide players into small groups. Give each group a paper bag filled with 5 or 6 everyday objects. You may or may not give the groups the same objects. The task for each group is to incorporate their objects into a short skit.

The Three Wizards (also known as "Dr. Know it All")

Description: The goal of this activity is for players to work together to come up with an answer to any question.

Directions: Ask for three volunteers. Together they become "The Three Wizards" or Dr. Know it All, and can answer any question asked. Each wizard (or part of the doctor) can only respond with one word at a time. If the first wizard begins the answer with "Because," the second wizard links his/her word to the first and the third wizard to the second. This panel of three must connect the words so that one complete statement is made in answering the question. For example, if the question asked is "Why is the earth round?", the dialogue might go as follows:

> 1st player: "Because..."
> 2nd player: "if..."
> 3rd player: "it..."
> 1st player: "wasn't..."
> 2nd player: "round..."
> 3rd player: "then..."
> 1st player: "it..."
> 2nd player: "couldn't..."
> 3rd player: "revolve..."
> 1st player: "around..."
> 2nd player: "the..."
> 3rd player: "sun."

The answer does not have to make sense as long as it is a complete statement. Ask group members to participate in questioning The Three Wizards. After some time, switch players and let others be The Three Wizards.

Let It All Hang Out

Description: Encourages players to get in touch with their inner feelings and express emotions.

Directions: Have everyone form a circle and face outward from the center. Name an emotion and ask players to react to it as if they were feeling that particular emotion at this particular time. Give them a while to play it out, then go on to the next emotion.

Show Me How You Feel Game

Description: Players connect with their (relatively) simple emotions.

Directions: This is a pantomime game in which participants are asked in turn to silently (through facial expressions and body gestures) express how they might feel in one of the situations characterized below:

Show me how you feel…

- when your stomach hurts
- when the sun is shining
- when you are eating ice cream
- when the nurse gives you a shot
- when your arm hurts
- when you are outside playing
- when a parent who is not living with you makes a visit
- when you are allowed to leave the hospital

Symphony of Emotions in Music

Description: The goals are for people to work together, to express emotions and to pay attention to the "conductor."

Directions: This can be played two ways. One option is to divide the group into smaller groups and ask each group to choose an emotion and an accompanying sound. The other option is to use the entire group, asking each member choose an emotion and an accompanying sound that describes the feeling. The facilitator acts as the conductor and creates a symphony. As the conductor points to each individual (or small group), the player(s) express the sound. After all individuals (or groups) have demonstrated their sounds, the conductor uses these sounds to create a symphony as if they were instruments in an orchestra. Everyone must pay close attention to the conductor in order to: start and stop on cue, increase or decrease volume or speed up/slow down the pace. Later the group can guess what emotions were being portrayed. After a demonstration the facilitator asks for volunteers to take turns acting as conductor.

Additional Theater Games

Instant Replay
Description: A name game commonly used as an ice breaker with a new group.
Directions: Have players form one large circle. Each person will have an opportunity to introduce him/herself to the rest of the group. Each player will choose a unique walk or movement which s/he will demonstrate by making the movement as s/he travels to the center of the circle. Once reaching the center of the circle s/he will introduce him/herself by name and return to his/her original spot. Once the player has returned to his/her spot, the rest of the group will mimic his/her actions and his/her name. Each player in turn does a different movement until the turn comes back to the first player.

Walk My Walk
Description: This is a good activity for identifying characteristics of people and translating them into movements.
Directions: Have players stand in a circle with plenty of space in the middle. Discuss the ways many people walk and show a few examples. For instance, a spy might creep along on tiptoes while a fashion model walks with a studied, erect posture. Players select a role with a specific kind of walk. Some ideas are

- tightrope walker
- astronaut on the moon
- body builder
- infant learning to walk
- marching soldier
- tired person
- window washer on a ledge
- explorer at the North Pole
- circus clown
- ninety year old man

Each player walks across the circle several times as the group tries to guess his/her identity. When someone guesses correctly, the entire group imitates the walk, then forms into a circle again to view another walk.

Passing the Buck
Description: Another good warm-up activity which helps the mind to "wake up" — the focus is on being creative and thinking fast.
Directions: Have everyone stand in a circle. The "buck" is any object that can be tossed easily from player to player — a glove, a beanbag, a nerf or rubber ball. Toss the "buck" to a player in the circle. The person catching the "buck" must begin to tell a story — something made up on the spot. This player (the one beginning the story) can start out with the familiar, "Once upon a time," or can start the story in any other way s/he chooses. The player holding the buck tosses it to another player who must catch it and continue the story. The story can take any form as long as there is an attempt to connect it to the last player's contribution. Players must not break the flow of the story no matter how fast the buck is passed. Those who have the buck must speak — if only a few words — before they can toss the buck to another player.

Who Started the Motion?
Description: Sharpens observational skills and awareness of others through the attempt to detect subtle changes in group's movements.
Directions: Players are seated in a circle. One player is sent from the room while the others select a leader to start the motion. With the group already in motion, the player is called back into the room. S/he stands in the center of the circle and tries to discover the leader, whose function it is to make a motion — tapping foot, nodding head, moving hands, etc. — and to change the motion whenever s/he wishes. The other players copy the leader's motions and try to keep the center player from guessing the leader's iden-

tity. Instruct players beforehand to stay closely in sync with the leader's motions and watch the leader using peripheral vision in order to better mask the leader's identity. When the center player discovers the leader, two other players are chosen to take their places.

Outright Lie

Description: Uses the imagination and humor. A good warm-up activity.

Directions: Select a small object such as a key, a ring, a pencil or scissors. Players should be seated in a circle and pass the object from person to person. As the object is passed around the room, each player must come up with an incredible story or fantasy to tell to the rest of the group. For example, if a key is selected, the stories might sound like this: "This key unlocks a treasure worth more than Fort Knox, a treasure located at the bottom of the Mediterranean Sea." Or: "This key saved the life of a man when it stopped a bullet while he was fighting in a war." After everyone has finished, ask the group members which lie they enjoyed the most.

Who (or "Who Am I?") Game

Description: This is an activity that helps players deal with an unknown situation and think on their feet.

Directions: Seat players in a circle. One player leaves the room. The remaining group decides on a profession or an identity for the person who left. One player (the "informant") stands up and when the first person comes back into the room this player initiates a conversation with him/her. The informant relates to the returned player as if s/he had the profession or the identity that the group has chosen for him/her. The returned player must keep the conversation going and try to guess his/her own identity by the direction of the conversation. Everyone in the room knows his/her identity except this player. The questions and answers given in conversation by the informant shouldn't be too easy, but should give clues to the returned player's identity. When the player guesses his/her profession, the audience applauds to show their acknowledgment and approval.

Talk Show
Description: A more advanced version of the "Who Game."
Directions: Two players leave the room in order to choose two famous characters to portray. Characters can be from real life or fiction, alive or dead and should be familiar to all or most of the group members. It is usually helpful if the two have some common interest such as music, sports or politics so that they can carry on a conversation. The two players then rejoin the group and begin to have a conversation such as two famous people meeting on a television talk show might have. Warn players not to give each other away with names. The other players (audience) try to guess who the two are by interviewing them. Group members who want to guess the two characters' identities do not call out their names but ask a question directly related to their identities. For example, if one of the guesses of famous people is George Washington, the question might be, "Do you get splinters from your wooden teeth?" If the guess is wrong and the player is not George Washington, s/he might answer, "I don't have to use wooden teeth since my teeth are all real." The audience (group members) continue to ask questions until many people seem to know the identities of the character. The leader asks the audience who the characters are and how they arrived at their conclusions. Usually the group is in agreement, but occasionally a character could be one of several people, which makes for an interesting discussion. The game ends when the group asks the characters to reveal their identities.

Mirrors
Description: Helps focus attention and teaches players to be both leaders and followers.
Directions: Divide the group into pairs. Have partners face each other. One player leads by making simple, slow movements which his/her partner mirrors — they then reverse roles. May use props.

After 5 minutes seat everyone in a circle. Select two players. They decide secretly who will be doing the mirroring. While looking in the "mirror" the other player demonstrates a simple activity such as washing or dressing. The audience tries to determine who is the mirror of the other. The better the players are at concentrating their attention on each other, the more "in sync" they will be and the harder it will be for the audience to guess the mirror.

Ripples
Description: Resembles the "wave" done at sporting events.
Directions: Gather the group into a single line behind a person chosen to be the leader. The object of the game is for each group member to follow the movements of the person directly in front of him/her, rather than following the leader directly. The leader begins a motion that is passed down the line. If the leader raises his/her arm, the second person follows the leader, the third person follows the second and so on down the line. The leader does not walk around the room but rather moves arms and legs, bends, leans and so on, in place. After players have done this a few times, divide the group into two lines with two leaders facing each other. In this version the second leader mirrors the movements of the first leader, and the group members follow the movements as above. Tell the leaders when to switch roles. For the grand finale, divide players into four groups with four leaders facing each other in a big X pattern. Two leaders initiate moves while the other two leaders standing across from them follow (Leader C follows the movements of Leader A and Leader D follows Leader B, for instance). Their group members follow one another as before. This version can be accompanied by music to create spectacular dance performances.

Lip Sync
Description: A good activity for developing cooperation and teamwork.

Directions: Four people play at a time. Two are actors and two are "dubbers." The rest of the group is the audience. The two actors decide on a real life drama that includes two characters and a situation. For example:

- Two people on vacation when their car runs out of gas
- A person smoking a cigarette in a non-smoking area and a non-smoker
- A person in a restaurant who keeps changing his/her order and an impatient waiter
- A door-to-door sales representative trying to sell someone a kangaroo (or other unnecessary object)

The actors and the dubbers work out a very rough plot outline without actually deciding on the dialogue. The actors play out the performance in pantomime. Offstage (out of view), the dubbers fill in the words. As the performance progresses, the actors and dubbers eventually affect each other and spontaneous things begin to happen. Switch actors and dubbers frequently. Try to give everyone a chance to be an actor or dubber at least once.

Transformations
Description: Another team-building activity that requires cooperation without much time for discussion.
Directions: Divide the group into two teams. The object of the game is for players to form as quickly as possible into human representations of whatever you describe. Call out the name of an object. Team members then must arrange themselves into that shape. For example, if you say "helicopter," players must work out how they will link together into propellers, cockpit and landing gear. Other ideas for transformations are: suspension bridge, ship, cathedral, capitol dome, tree, waterfall, truck, bus or skyscraper.

Real Life Drama
Description: Develops storytelling ability and sequencing (telling a story with a beginning, middle and end).

Directions: Players sit in a circle on the floor and tell the most interesting, dramatic or scary thing that has happened to them, such as: getting lost, playing in an exciting ball game, rescuing an ailing bird or animal, being in an accident or riding in a parade. Set a one minute time limit on each player's story. After everyone has told a story, divide the group into smaller groups of five or six. Each group selects several elements from each person's story that can be combined into a short skit. Encourage imaginative combinations, such as picking up a baby bird while crossing the goal line for the winning touchdown. Each group takes a turn to perform its skit for the (other players) audience.

City or Country
Description: This is done as a pantomime skit.
Directions: Divide the group into two or three teams. Pass out one (already prepared) situation card to each team. These situations be located in either the city or the country. Examples include:

The City
- An older lady enters a crowded bus, makes her way to the back and rides downtown.
- A fire breaks out in a school building and a teacher evacuates the frightened children.
- An all-night diner.

The Country
- An array of flowers growing in the garden.
- Giraffes feeding on lower branches of trees are joined by a friendly group of elephants.
- An approaching storm.

Each team has five minutes to determine who will do what in an impromptu skit depicting their situation. After five minutes each group performs for the others and the audience guesses what the situation was.

Laugh It Up

Description: Pure fun and a good icebreaker.

Directions: Divide the group into two teams. One side is heads and the other tails. The leader flips a coin and allows it to land on the floor. If the coin comes up heads, the heads team begins laughing, trying to make the opposite team laugh or smile. Teams must have eye contact with one another. There should be a time limit, perhaps 3 minutes. The tails team must hold firm, not laughing or smiling. If players do laugh, they must join the other team. Once all the tails people (who laugh) have joined the other side, and time is up, the coin is tossed once again. The game is over when everyone is on one side.

Pantomime

Description: Players try to convey a situation with pantomime (movements, gestures, facial expressions, etc.). No speaking is allowed. The audience must guess the situation from the pantomime. Everyone should have a turn acting out a situation. This can be played in teams keeping track of the time required to convey the situation. The following are examples of possible situations:

- Eating a banana
- Playing the violin
- Playing tennis
- Playing croquet
- Watching a tennis game
- Swatting a bothersome mosquito
- Walking a tightrope
- Juggling
- Putting on stockings
- A man shaving his beard
- Putting on a girdle
- Putting hair up in curlers
- Putting on lipstick
- Burping a baby
- Playing a trombone
- Conducting an orchestra
- Rowing a boat
- Paddling a canoe
- Doing the waltz
- Putting on nail polish
- Eating a watermelon at a picnic
- Typing on a typewriter
- Pitching a baseball

- Hanging clothes on a clothesline
- Milking a cow
- Policeman directing traffic
- Doing the hula
- Tying a necktie
- Washing clothes on a washboard
- Playing a harp
- Casting and catching a fish
- Shoveling snow
- Going to the dentist
- Putting a worm on a fish hook
- "Hear no evil, see no evil, speak no evil"
- Playing the bass drum, cymbals, triangle, etc.
- Voting in an election
- Threading a needle
- Making pancakes
- Getting ready to be married
- Hammering a nail into a stubborn piece of wood
- Listening to a dull minister in church
- Watching a horror movie
- Square dancing
- Toasting marshmallows over a campfire
- Playing in a craps game for a million dollars
- Doing a sailor's hornpipe
- Playing a piano dramatically in a concert

Group Hug

Description: A "good feelings" and group solidarity activity/closure to a theater session.

Directions: Have the entire group stand in a circle holding hands. Have the group step back until arms are extended out fully. Have group walk to the center of the circle (slowly) never breaking grip with each other. Return the group to the larger circle (stepping back slowly). Then have everyone race to the center, not breaking the grip. Finally gather the group together, arms around each other (group hug) and have them share what they may have learned from the session.

10

Drama

Drama therapy is a general term which encompasses three therapeutic techniques — Role Playing, Sociodrama and Psycho-drama — all of which are based on the principle that acting out situations can induce behavioral and/or psychological change in a person. Drama, according to Webster's dictionary, is "a state, situation or series of events involving interesting or intense conflict of forces." Drama is life in microcosm, action and reaction.

Therapists who choose to use the techniques of drama as a therapeutic modality should be aware of the purpose of each type, from problem-oriented role playing to (potentially) emotionally charged psychodrama. This will enable them to engage their clients at an appropriate level of dramatic intensity.

Role Playing

Role playing evolved from psychodrama but is a less emotion-ally intense experience. It is a vehicle for assisting clients to replay upsetting interactions with friends or family members, to practice social skills or experiment with new behaviors, or to confront peo-ple with whom they are angry. Real life issues can be explored in a safe environment. Role playing is problem oriented, one of its goals being to work out alternative and more effective approaches to identified problems. Another goal is to *change* behavior rather than to explore the psychodynamics of behavior (e.g., Why do I do this?). Since a primary aspect of this process is learning new behaviors, it is important for clients to receive feedback on the effectiveness of the behaviors practiced. Clients can continue to practice these behaviors until they are satisfied with them or until their anxiety is manageable.

Guidelines for the Use of Role Playing

Role playing is effective:

- Whenever the therapist wants to allow group members to be able to see themselves as others see them.
- When the group needs a change of pace from the activity or method currently being used to promote individual or group growth.
- Especially with couples, siblings, co-workers or for other relationships where problems in relating have developed.
- As a good technique for enabling us to laugh at ourselves and get out of the "drama" of life and its ruts.

The Setting

Chairs for the group are arranged in a circle. Depending on the nature of the role play, one or more chairs may also be placed in the middle of the circle. Items such as foam sticks, batakas or pillows may be made available for clients who need to vent feelings.

Warm Up: The Process of Selecting a Protagonist

From the standpoint of creating a positive learning experience, it is important to choose a group member who would benefit from assuming the role of protagonist. Evaluating information obtained from the following warm-up questions and considerations can help in making a choice.

Warm-up questions for the group:
- If you had a quarter who would you call and what would you say?
- What person do you have unfinished business with?
- The empty chair is you. What do you think about when you see that empty chair and what do you have to say to it?

Considerations:
- Generally, the protagonist should be picked by the amount of emotional affect exhibited in the warm-up.
- Avoid involving a reluctant protagonist.
- A protagonist who expresses a willingness to work should be considered.
- With an ongoing group you may choose to ask them who would like to work today and then have the group select from the situations offered or suggested.
- When in doubt wait and be patient. Perhaps even extend the warm-up period. There may be times when the whole session may become a warm-up activity.

Purposes of the Action
- To stimulate change: If an individual experiences him/herself acting in a spontaneous and creative manner in relation to others, and experiences others as accepting and giving, this person will tend to develop new perceptions of him/herself and his/her universe. This can have a beneficial effect on all aspects of life. The spontaneity of the action disrupts old patterns of behavior and can create an appropriate response to a new situation or a new response to an old situation.
- To provide alternatives within the context of a life situation.

- To allow the protagonist to play act a situation in a non-threatening environment. A supportive, non-judgmental atmosphere is important.

Selection and Use of the Double

This is the first step to take after selecting a protagonist. A "double" is a person whose function is to take on some aspect of personality or behavior for the protagonist. Determine who should play this role using one of the following methods:

- Ask the protagonist if s/he can choose someone in the group who knows him/her well enough to be able to help him/her.
- Ask the group if there is someone who identifies enough with the situation to serve as a double.

Roles of the Double

The double:

- may provide support or may be a mirror for the protagonist. S/he may also express thoughts and feelings the protagonist is unwilling to share.
- represents opposing viewpoints for the protagonist to consider.
- takes clues from the director.
- should try to imitate and try to get in touch with the feelings and thoughts of the protagonist.
- speaks for the protagonist rather than for him/herself.

The protagonist may disagree with the double at any time. The director may need to check back with the protagonist throughout the action to make sure that s/he remembers that this is an option. More than one double may be used. The following offers a deeper look at two techniques used by a double:

Mirror by the Double

One of the purposes of the double is to project an image through which the protagonist can see him/herself. For example, if the protagonist is expressing to a parent the fact that the parent never listens to what s/he says, the double may say, in the same intonation as the protagonist, "You never listen to what I say and how I feel!" This allows the protagonist to see and hear how the parent might perceive this statement. It adds another dimension, self-perception, to the reality of the situation.

Role Reversal in Role Playing

Role reversal gives the protagonist the opportunity to see and feel what it's like to be in "someone else's shoes." It helps the protagonist to become aware of the perceptions and views other than his/her own. It also introduces another person (besides the protagonist) into the scene for the protagonist to relate to.

The Role Play in Action

Any or all of these three techniques (double, mirror and role reversal) may be used within the role play period. The action may be set in the past, present, future or in fantasy.

Sharing Reactions

This is the *only* time that the whole group may participate, by sharing how they identified with the protagonist in the action. No interpretations are allowed but first-hand identifications and heart-felt responses are encouraged.

Closing

The closing is designed to fulfill two important functions:
- to provide support for the protagonist and thank him/her for his/her efforts.

- to provide the group with the opportunity to share supportive feelings with each other (e.g., applause, verbalizing, a group hug).

Life Situations Adaptable for Role Playing

The following section contains ideas for role playing. It is organized into two sections, the first containing general ideas for role playing social skills, followed by a group of more specific situations.

Personal Relationships (Friends, Relatives, Neighbors)

Giving and receiving compliments:
- being told that you did a good job
- telling someone that you like the way…
- complimenting another person on his/her hair, clothing, style, etc.

Stating feelings directly:
- finding something to be the focus of your life work and assuming your parent(s) disapprove
- anger towards someone who didn't keep a secret
- disappointment at a canceled date
- a friend continually being late
- stating fear about a situation
- needing more independence from family

Saying "NO!"
- to food not on your diet
- to an invitation
- to using drugs/alcohol
- to sexual involvement

- to a family gathering
- to someone smoking in your house
- to someone wanting to cheat off your exam

Asking for:
- support
- help
- time to spend with someone
- confidentiality

Telling someone about your:
- lack of interest in a love relationship
- disappointment in a relationship
- job loss
- serious health situation
- serious financial situation
- issues with in-laws
- separation or divorce

Defining/explaining to a five year old:
- the concept of "disability"
- the concept of "death"
- the concept of "divorce"
- the concept of "God"

Work Related Issues
- Job interview
- Termination interview (initiated by you)
- Termination interview (initiated by your boss)
- Difficulties with co-workers and:
  - smoking
  - drinking
  - covering for them (e.g., their mistakes or absences)

- competition for promotion
- Asking for assistance (feeling overworked)
- Dealing with authority figures (supervisor or boss)
- Dealing with social/sexual situations in the workplace
- Dealing with discrimination:
  - sexual
  - racial
  - disability related
  - social
  - age
  - professional advancement

Client/Therapist Relationships

Group members take on the roles required. Dealing with:
- "You are paid to care about us"
- Client flirting/asking for phone number
- Motivating a client
- A member of another discipline questioning what you are doing with a patient and the importance of your intervention

Risking Possible Rejection

- Your niece/nephew/son/daughter/someone you love very much and to whom you always tell the truth as you know it, wants to try out for a school play but is afraid s/he won't get the part.
- Your niece/nephew/son/daughter/someone you love very much wants to have a birthday party. She wants to invite some new friends but is concerned that they might not come.

Being Spontaneous

- Your best friend in the world wins a trip to Mexico and wants you to go; it would mean missing one week of school.

Creating Balance in Your Life

- Last weekend you spent the whole time playing and having fun, then felt completely guilty for not studying or "accomplishing anything constructive." The weekend before that you spent the whole time studying, washing clothes, cleaning house, etc. and resented not doing anything fun. However, this weekend...
- You are studying for a test that you must do well on the next day. Your friend calls you up with extra tickets to a concert. You've been eager to go to it, but unable to get tickets. You are not prepared for the test. What do you do?

Confrontation

- Your co-worker is on drugs. You are always covering up for him/her because s/he is often late. Your boss knows that there is a problem but wants the co-workers to work it out between them. How do you confront this person? Also, this person denies his/her problem.

Acceptance and Assertion

- You are winning an award. It is a great honor. What is it for?
- Someone crowds in front of you at the store/grabs the last copy of a book out of your hands/tries to talk you out of a purchase so that s/he can have it.
- Issues with authority/institutions, e.g., doctors or salespeople. For example, you have a feeling that you've been given too strong a prescription by your doctor.
- Disagreeing with a police officer (e.g., disputing whether you deserve a ticket).
- Being dissatisfied with:
  - a service done on your car.
  - your landlord.

- A person cuts ahead of you in line with two people ahead. The others don't say any thing. Would you?
- You take yourself out to a nice restaurant. You feel that you deserve something nice and love going out to eat. It doesn't matter that you are alone; in fact you're happy to have some private time. The waiter seats you close to the kitchen at a small table where you are invisible to others. In addition, you are not receiving appropriate service.
- You've had a new roommate for the past 3 months. She is now 5 days late with the rent. She just recently became unemployed and she is also ill with some flu-like symptoms that have lasted a week. She has made no attempt to borrow the money and just assumes you'll cover her rent. You confront her on the issue and she says she is too sick to talk about it. How do you react?
- Your boyfriend has recently started bringing up his old girl friend's name. Although it seems harmless, you know that there is still a strong bond between them. What do you do?
- You have been making dinner for your friend/lover and s/he was expected at 7:30 p.m. The table is set. It is already 8 p.m. and your guest has not arrived. An hour later the person arrives. This is not the first time you have found yourself waiting for this person. What do you do?
- A child has a pet guinea pig which the mother insists must be kept caged. The child is caught having let the little animal out to run loose in his/her room. There is a scene between mother and child involving the idea of caging/not following through on an agreement.
- A young woman comes home from an exciting event (a party, a drama class, a dance class) and is behaving in a spirited, noisy way. Her home, however, is a quiet place where one person is studying and another is watching TV. It is clear that her excitement and animated behavior are not welcome.
- You told a friend a personally embarrassing secret and the next morning another friend calls to console you.

- You have had a crush on a good friend who has been unavailable for the past few years. S/he has recently broken up with his/her significant other. You are still interested. What do you do?
- Someone you are intimately involved with asks you personal details about your past. You have been burned before by being completely honest. How do you respond?
- You are invited to a party by a new friend you met in one of your classes. You don't know anyone else who is going to the party, which is on Friday night. You usually spend Friday nights at home, watching TV or studying. You tell your friend...
- A grown daughter is trying to care for her elderly mother at home. The mother is very dependent and demanding. The daughter has not had any relief from her duties in quite a long time. As she tries to relax with a book, the mother calls out two rooms away for companionship.
- Michael, aged 33, is going to LA to visit his parents who have been retired for a couple of years now. Since retirement his father has been drinking more than he used to. Both of his parents are strong followers of the Protestant work ethic and used to work long hours in their family owned and run business. They sold the business at a profit in order to retire. When Michael arrives, his father has not returned yet from the golf club so Michael decides to disclose his concerns to his mother. She becomes angry at Michael for implying that his father has some sort of a "problem." Their conversation ends when Michael's father enters, returning from having "a few with the boys at the club."
- John, aged 43, is married to Linda, aged 36. They have been married for four years and are both satisfied with their relationship. While they are having dinner, Linda announces that she is interested in having a child. Taken by surprise, John announces firmly that he has no interest in going through that with her. When they first married, Linda was wrapped up in her career

and didn't think she wanted to have children. Now, as she hears her biological clock ticking, she has discovered that she has different feelings about the matter. Linda is disappointed in John's reaction; John is shocked and in a quandary at what he feels is Linda's change of heart.

- A divorced mother is at home cleaning on a Sunday afternoon. While picking up clothes off the floor in the room of her only daughter, who is aged 14 1/2, she finds her daughter's diary lying open to a recent entry. She reads the diary and discovers that her daughter is experimenting with cocaine and alcohol. The mother becomes enraged and is also frightened. She herself is an alcoholic who has been sober and in recovery for five years. Her daughter is aware of this and used to go to Ala-Teen meetings but has lost interest and refused to go this last year.

- Your newly single mother is going out on a date and you don't like the man.

- A friend suggests going to the movies and out to dinner. S/he wants to see a horror film and eat Mexican food. You would rather see a comedy and eat Chinese food, but every time you've gone out together, you've given in and have done what your friend wanted. This time however....

Additional Role Play Situations

- Somebody cuts right in front of you on the highway and proceeds to drive ten miles under the speed limit.

- You're at a party and your best friend is about to try cocaine.

- You're a baby sitter. You're not supposed to have boyfriends over. Your boyfriend calls and wants to come over.

- You're at a very busy restaurant and the waitress is already impatient. She brings you a meal that looks good but isn't what you ordered. She's about to walk away.

- You're at a party and some nerd persists in asking you to dance. You've politely tried everything to give him the message. You're now a little irritated… here he comes again. What do you do?

- You're at a dinner party and you're not able to eat what's served.
- You have a pot luck dinner and everyone brings dessert.
- You're late for an exam. On your way to class you see some guy drop his little black book. He doesn't realize he's dropped it and keeps walking. He's about 100 yards away.
- Your neighbor plays loud music every Saturday morning at 8 a.m. You worked until 3 a.m. Friday night.
- You're at a wedding party and they're passing a jug of wine around the table as a ritual toast. The wine is coming your way when you notice that the guy next to you has a cold sore on his lip.
- You've arrived in town just two days before your best friend's wedding. You hate the bridesmaids' dresses she had raved about over the phone. They're the wrong fit and the wrong color.

Sociodrama

This is a form of dramatic enactment which aims at clarifying *group* themes rather than focusing on the problems of one individual. Although an individual may participate as the protagonist in the sociodrama, characterization is based on a *type* of person rather than on any one individual. Sociodrama borrows many of the techniques of psychodrama (see next section) but the focus is always on creating or approximating real-life situations which concern the group as a whole. The goal of sociodrama is to help group members who share similar problems by exploring these problems together. Examples of sociodrama include the enactment of such situations as:

- A youth in a transition home seeing his/her parents for the first time since leaving the home environment.
- An alcoholic in a recovery program going to his/her first social event during recovery.
- An adult in a support group confronting an abusive situation.
- A group of residents in a nursing home confronting the nursing home administrator about a foul-mouthed aide.
- A group of female co-workers approaching the personnel manager about a male co-worker who belittles them.

Psychodrama

Psychodrama was developed by Jacob Moreno, MD in the 1920's. The primary characteristic which distinguishes psychodrama from other forms of drama therapy is that it is an exploration of one individual's internal conflicts. It focuses on the intrapsychic (internal) rather than the social (external) dimension. In psychodrama, the individual who is the main character (the protagonist) explores a conflict through an enactment that enables him/her to watch and engage in an inner drama as it becomes visible and tangible. The psychodrama may shift among the many facets of a protagonist's life — from his/her past to the present or future and back again. This technique usually focuses on relatively deep emotional issues, such as childhood traumas or painful memories, in order to uncover the origins of unresolved internal conflicts. Psychodrama is a method of action which makes conflicts available to people in a safe setting. This permits them to examine relationships in the present or re-examine past relationships which they consider relevant to the present, and to experiment with possible changes for the future.

In view of these two goals (examining the past and experimenting with change), psychodrama is often a two phase process. In the first phase, *re-enacting*, the core problem or frustration scene is acted out. Ideally the protagonist will experience catharsis (a profound emotion release) or fresh insight into a past problem in this phase. This is followed by the *correcting* or *retraining* phase. The protagonist corrects the negative scene by acting out a positive one that *s/he* delineates (Yablonsky, 1976). The following section describes the elements that comprise the first (*re-enacting*) phase of the psychodrama. The second phase (*retraining*) uses the same structure to replay a scene, but when it immediately follows the first phase, the warm-up may be omitted and only a short closure may be necessary.

Elements of Psychodrama

In psychodrama there is a ritualistic set of elements that help provide a structure for emotional release and discovery. These elements are the warm-up, enactment and re-enactment, catharsis-movement-emotional insight, closure of individual drama, sharing integrative process and closure of the group.

Warm-up

Warm-up techniques focus on spontaneity and interaction among group members in order to lessen inhibitions and prepare the group for the enactment. Group dynamics are revealed. (Who is included/excluded? Who identifies with whom?) The group is allowed to experience its own power, while the therapist balances the group needs against his/her own agenda for the group. During this period themes are also developing and the choices of protagonist and audience are becoming established.

Enactment and Re-enactment

Once the protagonist is chosen, s/he sets the scene and chooses roles for the enactment. The director now employs the techniques of psychodrama to begin the process. These techniques are meant to facilitate the protagonist's ability to experience feelings throughout the scene.

Catharsis — Movement — Emotional Insight

For Moreno, the concept of catharsis was an important aspect of psychodrama. The protagonist undergoes a self-purging and the audience witnesses and engages in an emotional experience. Psychodrama thus draws on both the power of the stage and of religious ritual (Moreno in Emunah, 1994). The catharsis and emotional insight is a turning point that takes place near the closure of the enactment. Catharsis may involve regression in the service of the ego, but it is *not* an acting out to avoid a painful memory, it is a reprocessing of memory.

Closure of Individual Drama

The timing of closure is a therapeutic judgment. When the director feels that the drama is coming to a close, s/he may say, "How do you want to end this?" In addition to the protagonist, the director must also consider the group's investment in the enactment. At times, when a particular scene affects the group strongly, it may be difficult to continue the scene (e.g., themes of suicide, homicidal ideation, drug use). It is important to find out the group's feelings in order to determine what to do next. The director may say something like, "It looks like everyone felt strongly about what went on. Try finishing this sentence, 'What touched me was _____.'" The answers may give information for further work.

Sharing Integrative Process

This is the only time the whole group can participate by sharing how they felt. No interpretations are allowed — the group should also be discouraged from just saying what they saw the players doing. During the sharing statements following the enactment, the audience makes evident their identification with the protagonist. Most experience common or universal feelings about what took place. The director may check out impressions of the audience. For example the director may ask a member of the audience, "You seemed tense during the scene, did you feel tense? Did the scene have an impact on you?" The director will help the group identify the similarities and differences in feelings and experience of group members. Through the sharing, the director tries to create opportunities to develop empathy and a trusting milieu.

Closure of Group

The closing of action provides support for the protagonist and thanks him/her for his/her efforts. It is also the time to give the group the opportunity to share supportive feelings with each other (e.g., applause, verbalizing or group hug).

At closure the group may acknowledge that it will (in a new drama) further explore an area or examine a theme that emerged.

Techniques of Psychodrama

Warm-up Techniques

These techniques have as their aim the facilitation of spontaneity which helps lessen emotional inhibition in group members. Thematic content is often obtained through warm-ups and may lead to the development of a psychodrama.

Magic Shop

Values are exchanged by barter. A hope, wish, aspiration or personal quality is obtained by exchanging another personal quality for it. One after another, members of the group volunteer to enter the magic shop in quest of a dream, quality or aspiration. The barter compels the subject to judge the relative value of the qualities and his/her desire for them. A written exchange may reinforce the interaction. The audience may be asked to assist the shopkeeper or to comment on the deal being arranged. A sample dialogue might be

Customer: "I would like to buy some time for myself."

Shopkeeper: "I have that over here in aisle two. What can you trade?"

Customer: "Well, I'll trade some ambition to get some time for myself."

Shopkeeper: "I thought you valued your ambition — that achieving was what made your life meaningful. Are you sure you are ready to give up your ambition?"

Customer: "I think that I am getting sick from not having time for myself. Maybe I can keep some of my ambition in this bottle until I need it and give the rest to you."

Empty Chair

Here the audience is told to imagine a person sitting in an empty chair which is before them. They are told to picture, for example, the person's dress, appearance and posture. Each member then tells of the person that s/he projected to be in the chair. This frequently yields thematic content leading to a psychodrama.

One Wish

Group members are asked to state what they would wish for if a magic genie could grant them only one wish. For example, a client might wish for "fears and anxieties to melt away." This wish could lead to a psychodrama about what life would be like without fear and anxieties.

One Day to Relive

Group members are asked to choose one day that they would like to relive if they were given the opportunity to do so.

Who Would You Like to Be?

Group members are asked, "Who would you rather be?" This question, used in an enactment, might provide a good opportunity for role reversal, enabling the protagonist to become the person s/he wishes to be.

Coloring Book
Members are asked to draw their own worlds, the imaginary materials being a crayon and blank pages. "What would you draw on the first page? On the second page?" and so on.

Non-Verbal Techniques
The group consents to interact with one another for a fixed period of time during which the use of words is forbidden. Members are encouraged to express anything they feel at the moment using movement of any body part(s) (e.g., hand gestures) as the mode of expression. They may use the physical setting (e.g., chairs) in any way but must respect the one rule — no words. Rich material develops as patterns of reaction come into relief against the background of silence.

Thematic Psychodramatic Techniques
These techniques consist of thematic suggestions presented to the group.

Future Projection
The protagonist picks a point in time and projects him/herself into the future, enacting a situation that s/he thinks will come about, or one that may actually be expected to come about, e.g., an interview for a job, a pending marriage or birth. Future time techniques requires that the protagonist imagines what life will be like "if."

Self-Realization
The protagonist enacts his/her hopes, plans and aspirations as s/he wishes them to be, not as s/he expects them to be.

Dream Representation

The protagonist enacts a dream instead of telling it. In a discussion with the director, the protagonist describes the dream, then auxiliary egos are selected from the group to take parts in the dream: to be the voices, objects or persons. The protagonist takes the position s/he usually has when sleeping and then proceeds to enact the dream. In the retraining phase, the protagonist is told that s/he can change the dream in any way s/he wishes.

Hallucinatory Psychodrama

The protagonist enacts the hallucinations and delusions s/he is experiencing. S/he portrays the different aspects of the hallucination: the voices, sounds or visions. Auxiliary egos may be called upon to enact the various hallucinatory phenomena so that the protagonist can interact with them and thereby put them to a reality test. The aim is that through the enactment and interaction within the psychodrama, the subject will begin to have some control over his/her hallucinations.

Behind Your Back

Here the protagonist turns his/her back to the rest of the group. The group is told to imagine that the protagonist is not present. Each participant shares feelings towards the protagonist. This segment is followed by a discussion. The protagonist is then "brought back into the room" and the discussion continues.

Variation: Have the group turn its back on the protagonist, who then makes an honest statement about his/her feelings towards each group member.

These techniques are useful in group therapy situations as they provide a means of clarifying and resolving interpersonal difficulties among group members.

Facilitative Techniques Within a Psychodrama

Once a thematic structure has been established (see above), this group of techniques is aimed at facilitating catharsis, insight and role perception within the psychodrama.

Double

In this technique the protagonist plays him/herself. An auxiliary ego, usually a staff member, is asked to also represent the protagonist, e.g., to assume the same emotional and physical positions and therefore to assume the identity of the protagonist. The double then may express feelings, thoughts, opinions and reactions which the protagonist cannot or will not voice him/herself.

Multiple Double

The protagonist plays him/herself, and several auxiliary egos play parts of the protagonist. This technique may aid in clarifying an issue or restructuring ambivalence about a person or situation, and may facilitate catharsis.

Mirror for Expression

If a protagonist is inhibited to the point of immobilization so that s/he cannot represent him/herself in word or action, an auxiliary ego may be chosen (by the protagonist or director) to be a "mirror" of the protagonist's movements and speech. Such a representation or mirroring would be under the direction of the protagonist who would inform, correct or change the mirror's psychodramatic representation.

Role Reversal in Psychodrama

This technique has two major functions.
1. Role reversal may occur during a scene in order to aid the auxiliary ego in accurately enacting the role assigned to him/her by the protagonist. Here, the reversal is of short duration but is long enough to provide clues to the auxiliary ego to create a more accurate representation of the role.

2. Role reversal is especially useful in the learning or retraining phase of the process. Through reversal of roles, the protagonist is given the opportunity to experience the feelings of the "other" in an interpersonal situation. Moreno (1985) states, "the function of role reversal is to increase role perception."

Physical Elevation

In order to promote full expression of feelings toward an "other" (usually an authority figure) in a psychodramatic scene, the protagonist can be physically elevated by standing on a chair, stool or table and interacting with the "other." Frequently, this produces an authoritativeness on the part of the protagonist which can be difficult to attain using other techniques.

11

Laughter and Clowning

Too often, when someone has an illness or disability, it is hard for that individual to look beyond the crisis and discomfort. This micro-focused vision produces an imbalance. To help the patient achieve a balance again, a balance of recognizing all that is in his/her world, both the good and the bad, humor is often used. Laughter is an important component of wellness. This chapter will look at the difference of laughing with instead of at someone and the treatment benefits of laughter.

One of the ways to promote laughter is with clowning activities. A clown is an entertainer who uses antics, jokes and tricks to help produce a happy, lighthearted mood. If clowning is the activity then smiles and laughter are the obvious signs of the desired outcome. The second part of the chapter will provide information on running clown activities as one of the ways to promote healthy laughter.

Laughing

Laughing with someone tends to be based on mutual respect and caring for the other. The laughter develops empathy between groups, giving each a greater confidence. This brings individuals closer together, providing support and emotional nourishment through amusement. Healthy laughter breaks down emotional barriers instead of creating or reinforcing them. Some individuals (including clowns) may choose to place themselves at the butt of their own jokes. This is done in such a way as to bring joy and esteem to all involved, including the teller of the joke. The person who affords a healthy laugh at himself/herself invites other people to laugh and feel more at ease.

Laughing at others tends to be based on contempt and insensitivity toward others. This type of laughter divides people and destroys confidence. This division excludes some people, offends others and tends to reinforce negative stereotypes by singling out individuals or groups. When a person doesn't have a choice about being the butt of a joke, hurt feelings develop and grow, even if the teller of the sarcastic joke is the butt of the joke. This type of laughter is often abusive in nature and chills any hope of developing a closer, open group.

Benefits of Laughter

There are many health benefits associated with laughter. Using laughter as part of a therapeutic intervention helps promote physical well-being, provides cognitive stimulation and feelings of social well-being, increases coping skills and helps increase the individual's subjective well-being.

The physical act of laughing allows the individual to exercise his/her lungs and chest muscles. This, in turn, helps stimulate the circulatory system. Laughter used on a regular basis helps the body to relax its muscles, lower the pulse rate and may even help lower blood pressure. Laughter also helps the individual cope with and control pain through increased production of endorphins (the body's naturally occurring pain killer). The distraction from pain caused by laughter also goes a long way toward the successful coping with pain. It is hard to hold strongly to anxiety, fear, tension and/or anger when you are laughing so hard you are crying.

Laughter not only promotes better circulation by increasing blood and oxygen flow to the brain, it also encourages the individual to cope with adversity, think flexibly and achieve (and keep) mental health. Humor helps increase an individual's coping skills, deflating anger and helping ease stressful situations. Somewhat tongue-in-cheek Konrad Lorenz (1963) observed that "Barking dogs may occasionally bite, but laughing men hardly ever shoot. (p. 285)." Truly, laughter is one of the primary defenses in the human repertoire for coping with and adapting to stress and trauma. Valiant (1977) conducted a study using a group of healthy men to identify mature coping mechanisms. Humor was one of the five coping mechanisms identified through his study.

Humor also helps social interactions. Humans are social creatures. Being in close proximity to others tends to produce tension, divide relationships, and necessitate coping with anti-social acts by others. Humor provides one of the mechanism for coping with the results of being close to others. Usually, joyful and humorous interactions between two individuals are indicators of a close and healthy relationship.

Clowning Activities[6]

Since clowning uses antics, jokes and tricks to help produce a happy, lighthearted mood and smiles and laughter are the obvious signs of the desired outcome, clowning makes sense as a therapy

---

[6] The information for this section was furnished by "Make*A*Circus" of San Francisco, CA, an organization which conducts clown therapy workshops for a wide variety of facilities.

tool. The staff of "Make*A*Circus" generally use the following protocol when working with groups:

Meet with staff to prepare for the session
Topics of discussion include:
- Status of clients
- Staff availability
- Lessons to accomplish

Begin session by creating clear parameters to insure safety
- Within the safety parameters instill acceptance and appreciation for each other's work.

Warm-up bodies and minds
- Explore within a safe environment.
- Begin the process of ensemble.
- Stimulate and support imagination and acceptance.
- Physically prepare the body and mind.
- Establish the process of "learning through imitation."
- Use clowning as a tool for assessment without embarrassing anyone.

Introduce and refine skills
- Learn to execute multi-step directions.
- Learn to work together in pairs.
- Continue to develop safe, controlled learning experiences.
- Develop specific fine and gross motor skills.

Allow all to experience the process
- Explore the ensemble process.
- Take risks.
- Support others.
- Stay within the rules of decorum.

Provide for a period of winding down and transition
- Relax.
- Redirect group focus to the next activity.

After class, meet with staff to evaluate and plan the next session

Clown Safety

Before starting our eight-to-ten week session, the Make*A*Circus staff meet with agency staff in order to familiarize themselves with procedures and safety concerns of the individual facility. We then incorporate the agency's rules into our programming. We are there to support the agency and will comply with staff decisions.

Basic Clowning Rules

There are three "NO" rules and three "YES" rules:

The "No's":
- NO sharp objects in pockets!
- NO teasing!
- NO flipping or tumbling without staff supervision!

The "YES's":
- YES...Listen!
- YES...Wait your turn!
- YES...Freeze like statues!

Extra Safety

On the day that we introduce "slaps and falls" we reintroduce the concept of the "Clown Oath."

I (clown name) promise never, never, never, never, never, never, never, ever, ever, never, ever, never, ever to hit or hurt another clown!

Hitting or hurting another clown is grounds for termination from the program.

Developing a Clown Program

Not all facilities will have access to clowns. Lisa De Vries, a recreational therapist in the Seattle area, retells how she started a clowning program to enhance her therapy program in a long term care facility.

As a recreational therapist, I am always in search of new ways to meet the needs of my clients. In a recent conversation on the topic of new programs, a colleague suggested that I add clown visits to the program at my facility. It was successful with her patients. I began the search for a clown who would volunteer to come to the facility where I worked. That was a long and fruitless process. I entertained the idea of going to clown school, but my administer was not willing to support the time or the money for the endeavor. That just left my staff and me to use our creativity to become clowns ourselves. We bought a book, found some costumes at a garage sale, practiced balloon animals and borrowed a popcorn maker, and the clowns were born.

Clowning is not an easy task. It takes a great deal of energy. People expect clowns to be funny and energetic. People expect clowns to make funny animals and dance to the music in their rooms and maybe even tell a joke. It was not easy, but we made ourselves up so it was difficult for patients to identify who we were. We spent one afternoon a month at the facility visiting, making balloon animals, dancing, laughing and even telling a joke or two. The results were amazing.

I saw patients in a long term care center open their eyes wide, smile, laugh and even speak, when those things were thought to be long gone for them. One patient in particular lifted her head when I touched her and she smiled and kissed my big red spongy nose. She let me hold her hand and dance with her in her chair. Patients where I worked looked forward to the visit of the clowns. We paid no attention to abilities or looks. We were the funny people who danced, laughed and made a balloon animal for everyone.

The benefits of clowning are great for a variety of patients. The clowns with color alone can provide new and exciting sensory stimulation. The clowns are like pets and children in health care. We are accepting and we have no history of making the patient do something they do not wish to do. We have never hurt a patient. Clowns are things of happy memories. And clowns can make patients laugh. Often times in health care, laughter is a forgotten commodity. Research has shown that part of physical health is mental health. Clowning is one way to improve mental health.

Not only is clowning beneficial to patients, it is beneficial to staff morale, family interaction and morale, and departmental recognition in your facility. Staff loved to see the clowns come. I can recall a number of staff commenting on patient response to our visits as clowns. They comment on how the patients seem to perk up as we walk down the halls. They also enjoy some popcorn or a balloon animal. Families love to see their family member interact in a new way. It is a time to have fun together in what can be a bad situation. When the clowns began to visit, it increased the amount of discussion about the department among staff and administration. It also increased the amount to time that was spent with each patient, as we visited every patient on an individual basis in that afternoon.

The benefits of clowning can be transferred to other populations of patients. I happen to work with long term care patients with a goal of sensory stimulation, social interaction and increased quality of life. But clowns can work in rehabilitation, oncology and general medical floors with some of the same goals and more. I have used my clowning skills to work with a rehabilitation patient on fine motor skills. He happened to be a clown in a local group. We made animals together after his stroke. It was beneficial for his fine motor skills, but it also engaged other patients on the unit who wanted to learn the skill or get an animal for a family member who would be visiting later.

As a recreational therapist, I have found that clowning has been one of the best therapy tools that I could every have chosen to learn. It works with a variety of patients, it meets many different needs and it makes the patient happy. It is far easier to refuse a therapist when it is time for treatment than it is to refuse a clown.

The one patient population where clowning may not work is young children. While we often associate children, the circus and characters such as Bozo the Clown as good matches, for children developmentally under the age of seven, the opposite may be true. Children who are in hospitals may see twenty to thirty health care professionals a day related to their treatment. Many of these professionals will prod, poke or otherwise cause pain while they are wearing funny blue cloth shoes, wearing which modify their faces and big, baggy coats. Often young children do not distinguish between medical staff and clowns, quickly reacting with tears and screams when any adult dressed thusly approaches. Also, young children explore the world by mouthing objects and rubber balloons are one of many objects which shouldn't go into the mouth. Balloon tricks using rubber balloons should not be shared with young children to reduce the chance of inhaling and choking on broken balloon pieces.

Clowning Resources

Books

Bolton, R. 1982. **Circus in a Suitcase**. Rowayton, CT: New Plays, Inc.

Burgess, H. 1990. **Circus Techniques: Juggling, Equilibristics, Vaulting**. New York, NY: Thomas Y. Crowell Co.

Cline, P. 1991. **Fools, Clowns and Jesters**. New York, NY: Simon & Schuster Children's.

Disher, M. W. 1979. **Clowns and Pantomime**. Stratford, NH: Ayer Co.

Grock (Adrian Wettach). 1931. **Life's a Lark.** Stratford, NH: Ayer Co.

Schechter, J. 1985. **Durov's Pig: Clowns, Politics and Theatre.** New York, NY: Theatre Communications Group.

Townsen, J. 1976. **Clowns**. New York, NY: Hawthorn Books.

Juggling Equipment

More Magic and Illusions
554 Boston Post Road
Milford, CT 06460
800-876-8484

Rob's Magic and Juggling Shop
3023 Central NE
Albuquerque, NM 87106
800-705-8425

Brian Dupe
25 Park Place
New York, NY 10007
212-619-2182

Make Up (Kryolan, Aquacolor)

Kryolan
132 Ninth St.
San Francisco, CA
415-863-9684

Clown Antics
38092 Hixford Place
Westland, MI 48185
313-721-3970

Special Effect Supply
543 W. 100 N. #3
Bountiful, UT 84010
801-298-9762
FAX: 801-298-9763

Lynch's Inc.
939 Howard
Dearborn, MI 48124
800-24-LYNCH

12

Music

Music therapy is the functional application of music to bring about changes in behavior. Music therapy focuses on:

- **Conceptual development** — learning basic concepts of music and musical language.
- **Body image and body awareness** — use of the body to express or match rhythm and melody, strengthening body image in the process.
- **Gross and fine motor skills** — rhythm and coordination (e.g., clapping, dancing, use of instruments).
- **Tactile discrimination** — music has texture, surfaces create music (e.g., shuffling feet across floor).
- **Auditory memory** — listening and remembering what is heard.
- **Auditory sequencing** — ordering, as in learning stanzas of a song, and time-order, as in learning when to sing and when to be quiet.
- **Socializing** — engaging with other members of a group.

concept dev. tactile
auditory seq. dev.
auditory memory
socialization

Main Goals and Focus of Treatment

One goal of music therapy is to enable the therapist to assess several areas of client's abilities. These areas include a client's perceptual motor skills, sensory motor level of functioning for both gross and fine motor skill, and whether his/her behavior is age-appropriate.

The treatment focus of music therapy may be on rehabilitating either an individual or providing benefit to a group. The musical activities also help the therapist work on improving clients' social skills and achieving age-appropriate behavior in an environment that is fun and creative. Music therapy is a "permissive" outlet — one which may be very effective for clients who have difficulties expressing their energies or emotions through other means.

Group Structure

Participants in a music therapy group usually sit in a circle on the floor. A circle has several advantages: it affords unity, eye contact, social interaction and sharing. The leader makes a statement which is then repeated around the circle. The statement identifies the task or area of development or sharing that is being stressed. For example, the task may be to create a rhythm that will be imitated by other members of the group. Activities take place in the center of the circle.

Chanting, singing and rhythm activities are the essence of the music therapy group. The group is highly structured — although leadership is passed around the circle and there is room for creativity, the therapist provides most of the encouragement, reassurance and support.

The Activity is Secondary to the Process

The following points are worth bearing in mind:

- Participants tend to remember what they *did* during a group rather than the fact that they could finally play a song together.
- There is rarely something concrete for them to take away with them; hopefully what they *have* taken has been internalized.
- Activities may differ but the way an individual member of the group approaches these activities will remain the same.
- Peer relationships, rejection issues and impulse control issues can be identified and worked on repeatedly; new behaviors can be practiced and/or old ones changed or modified.

There are two types of activities: individual and group.

Individual activities require the following skills:

- generating sounds
- generating movement
- sequencing
- concentrating on a task
- following instructions
- ability to sustain effort
- reacting appropriately to objects

Group activities also require the following:

- paying attention
- sharing
- understanding and setting boundaries
- interacting with others appropriately
- listening to others
- waiting for a turn
- cooperation
- ability to be the center of attention and to relinquish it
- ability to generate camaraderie

Activities might include:
- sing-a-longs
- Orff Schulwerk
- listening
- music and movements
- dance
- improvisation
- vocals
- instrument lessons
- guided imagery

The Orff Schulwerk Technique

Carl Orff created this technique in Germany during the 1920's. By the end of World War II it had made its way to the United States. Schulwerk literally translated means "school work," and was originally created to teach school children the fundamentals of music and creative expression. Hence the name "Orff Schulwerk." Clinically, Orff is a group process that respects individuality, provides an outlet for self-expression and creativity and ensures success for the participant.

Orff is a series of improvisations that move clients in a stepwise progression toward successful self-expression. In Orff, participants learn the power of creativity as it affects other members of the group. The activities are based on making a response in imitation of the model. This design develops the echo form or question-answer form. Leadership is passed around the circle and a sense of group ensemble starts to build.

Orff Schulwerk Rondos

Use the rondos below to work on concepts of rhythm and group interaction. Some, especially the interpersonal game rondos, provide non-threatening ways to express feelings that might be hard to express in normal conversation.

Name Game Rondos

Name game   (clap clap)
Name game   (clap clap)
Let's play   (clap clap)
A name game (clap clap)

Name game, name game,
What's your name
And what's your game?

One hand says, "How do you
    do?"
The other says, "Who are
    you?"

If a fruit for a name,
You had to take
What kind of choice
Would you make?

Names go up
*(use hand motions to indicate
    up and down)*
Names go down.
Play the way
your name sounds.

Interpersonal Game Rondos

Music, music in the air
Make some music
A friend can share.
*(pick an instrument and play it,
    then next person chooses an
    instrument to play with
    him/her)*

Anyone can be any shape they
    want to be
Anyone can be any shape they
    want to be
Big, tall, short, small
Anyone can be any shape they
    want to be
What can you be?

I've got my face,
I've got my hat.
I've got my body under that
How do I seem? How do I feel?
Look at me and see what's real.

Great big people
Stamp around,
Little tiny people
Touch the ground.

Tambourines, bells
Triangles and a gong
Now it's your turn
To make up a song.

It's late at night
And I'm as hungry as can be
When I get to the kitchen
What do I see?

If wishes and dreams
Could come true
This is what
I'd wish for you.

Rhythms are fun
Rhythms are free
Can you make
A rhythm for me?

You are you
If you were me
What would you do?

Whispers are nice
Whispers are fun
Pass one along
How far will it run?

Magic blob,
What can it be?
Make it into something
Then pass it to me.

Look out the window
See the sky
What do you feel?
What would you do
If you could fly?

When you feel low
Know what you can do?
Just say goodbye
To whatever is bugging you
What's got you?

Tee shirts and jeans
Tee shirts and jeans
What else do you wear
Besides Tee shirts and jeans?

The witch has an itch
The witch has an itch
Where, oh where,
Is the witch's itch?

Alike and different,
Alike and different,
We are both,
Alike and different.

Hey shadow, ho shadow
Show us what you do,
Hey shadow, ho shadow,
Show us what you do
We'll do the same as you.

Icka becca soda cracker
What a silly sound.
Icka becca soda cracker
Get up and move around.

Rondos with Props

Prop: shoe
Listen carefully to the shoe
Tell us what it says to you!

Prop: ball
Wall, ball
Where do you fall?

Prop: box
What's in the box,
What's in the box
Sweat socks, goldilocks
What's in the box?

Prop: broom
This is my broom
To sweep away
The things I don't like
In myself today.

Prop: magnet
This is my magnet
To bring to me
The things I like
And want to be.

Prop: pillow
Pillow, pillow
Stuffed with love
Release in me
My adventurous dove.

Prop: paper cup
Look what I found
It's small and round
Before I lose it
I'll show you how to use it.

Prop: bubbles
Bubbles, bubbles
In the air
Blow some bubbles
We all can share.

Prop: top
Spin, spin, spin till it stops
When it stops
I'll be on top.
(Group says: on top of what?)

Prop: wrapped box with bow
Boxes, boxes
Tied with bows
Show me how
Your present goes.

Prop: mask (blank paper plate)
This is my mask
My mask makes me glad
I like my mask
Because it's _____.

**Prop: wall made of card-
    board**
This is a wall, this is a wall
How can we get over it?
How can we get over it?
Once and for all?
Answer:
This is a wall, this is a wall
We can use a ladder
Once and for all.

Prop: stick, like a wand
*(Everyone helps to choose one
    animal. Touch person with
    "wand.")*
You are (name of animal, e.g.,
    baboon)
A baboon, A baboon
What do you do, baboon?
What do you do?

Prop: tambourine
This is a tambourine,
a tambourine, a tambourine,
this is a tambourine
what else could it be for?
Prop: key and tambourine

*(Two people, person A and
    person B)*
A: I'm the musical lock
B: I'm the musical key
A: To open the lock
you must do the same as me.
*(B imitates simple rhythms
    played by A on tambourine.
B then "opens" lock and chant
    is repeated with next per-
    son.)*

Prop: assorted hats
*Each participant chooses a
    hat, puts it on and takes on
    the role that the hat suggests
    (cowboy hat, police hat,
    veiled lady's hat, army hat,
    baseball cap, etc.). Partici-
    pant may then be interviewed
    by an "on the street re-
    porter" as the group chants:*
S/he walks right over
Pats the hat on his/her head
Walk up to the microphone
And this is what s/he said…

Projective Game Rondos
Who's that tapping at my window?
Who's that tapping at the door?
It's my _____ tapping at the window,
And my _____ tapping at the door.

When I was a little girl(boy), little girl, little girl
When I was a little girl, _____years old
(tell something that happened, for example)
My ice cream cone fell on the floor,
(repeat previous line)
My ice cream cone fell on the floor.
Bless My Soul.
(positive resolution)
My grandpa got another one, another one,
(repeat previous line)
My grandpa got another one, another one.
Bless My Soul.

Tok-a-dee *(hit knees twice)* Ko-dee *(clap hands twice)*
(Snap fingers on left hand twice and look to left then snap fingers on right hand twice and look to right.)
Tok-a-dee Ko-dee
Tok-a-dee Ko-dee
(Snap fingers on left hand twice and look to left then snap fingers on right hand twice and look to right.)
After you have established a rhythm, say the name of the person to your left and right as you snap your fingers. This process continues around the circle of participants. The tempo may be sped up or slowed down.

Additional Activities Using Music

The following activities range from those imposing the least amount of structure to those with the most structure:

Total Group Effort
Everyone begins playing the Orff Schulwerk instruments. The leader listens, finds a steady beat and plays it. The group repeats the pattern set up by the leader.

Play How You Feel and Title It

This activity may be done individually, in a group with each person taking a turn, or as a group. Express a feeling using the rhythm, volume and/or pace of the music.

Letting Go of Something

Players imagine something that they are trying to "let go of." It could be, for example, a worry, an angry feeling or a troubling thought. Individuals in the group play to express this "letting go" experience.

Conversations Between People

Two group members have a conversation using their instruments. You may add a third person (limit to three people so the observers can still follow the "conversation").

Creating a Musical Score

Divide the group into several small groups. Each group decides on symbols (which are then cut out of colored construction paper) for each of the musical instruments available to them. On a large piece of butcher paper they place the symbols and notes to create a musical score. Each person chooses an instrument, identifies the symbol that represents his/her instrument and plays the notes. One member needs to be the conductor.

Exploration

Sitting in a circle, the leader begins by playing a one beat sound. Others follow. Then the leader changes to two beats. See if the group can follow. Start gently, gradually become more aggressive, then gentle again…building to faster, fastest, then slowing down, to closure.

Rain

Group members sit in a circle, facing the center. Members close their eyes, pausing for a moment or two of quiet while getting ready to repeat the sound the person on his/her right will be making. All members keep their eyes closed and the rainstorm gets underway as the leader rubs his/her palms together, back and forth in a circular movement. The person to his/her left joins in, and then the next person to the left, and the next person, continuing on around the circle until everyone is rubbing palms and listening to the drizzling rain building in intensity. When the leader hears the drizzling sound being made by the person on his/her right, s/he starts snapping his/her fingers. One by one within the circle, finger snapping replaces palm rubbing and the sprinkling rain turns into a steady patter. When the snapping action has been picked up by everyone, the leader switches to hand clapping, then progresses to slapping thighs and finally stomping feet. Then the storm subsides, just in reverse of the way it grew: moving from foot stomping to thigh slapping, hand clapping, finger snapping and back to palm rubbing. If the group is having trouble hearing the changes, members can alert neighbors with a gentle nudge each time their movement switches from one action to the next.

13

Dance/Movement and Movement Exploration

These two modalities are not, despite the similarity of their names, interchangeable. Dance/movement therapy is much more concerned with the psychological implications of movement on and by the client, whereas movement exploration is just that: an exploration of the possibilities of movement through space.

Goals of Dance/Movement Therapy

Dance/Movement is a "statement of emotion expressed through movement." (Warren, 1984) Therapists who focus on dance/movement as therapy seek to correlate cognitive process, emotions and movement. The primary goal of dance/movement therapy is to assist clients in achieving a greater degree of body integration and awareness. Within this broad goal are three sets of goals which may be of greater importance to a given client population.

The first is *emotional:* movement also releases emotion. Through dance/movement therapy, clients may find a structure that will help them express overwhelming emotions, such as anger, fear

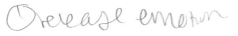
release emotion

and sadness. Dance/movement can enable them to work through conflict, tension and distortion (as in the case of those suffering from dyssynchrony, fragmentation, or catatonia). An increase in the ability to express oneself may correlate with an increased range of physical motion as well.

A second set of goals is *physical.* Dance/movement exercises can help clients experience control over impulsive, random behavior, such as manic ritualistic movement. A client can be taught to better integrate a range of movements, from spontaneous to coordinated (coming from either extreme, the infantile and impulsive or the mechanical). For the individual with physical challenges (e.g., cerebral palsy) dance/movement may help the client gain control over muscle spasms as part of a creative and relaxed experience. Dance/movement therapy can help strengthen a realistic sense of body image and perception of self (e.g., for patients with eating disorders).

Finally, the goals of dance/movement therapy may be *social.* Clients are given the opportunity to interact and share with others in a way which is non-verbal (through movement — as in "group rhythm," a way of responding and relating) and verbal (imagery). Dance/movement offers clients, especially more withdrawn individuals, a unique way to develop relationships with others and with their environment.

Assessment/Observation

Every movement in dance/movement therapy is seen as *adaptive* (a coping mechanism) and *expressive* (reflective of the individual). The following aspects and ranges of movement are observed, evaluated and worked with in dance/movement therapy:

Use of effort/presence
- shape of actions (away or toward body)
- use of body planes (vertical, horizontal, sagittal)

- attitudes toward space (direct to indirect)
- time (ranging from quick to sustained)
- force (strength to lightness)
- movement into space (directional and shaping motions)
- relationships between gesture (isolated body part) and posture (the activation of many parts in relation to each other)

Dance/Movement Activities

Body Warm Up
Group members are asked, "Where in your body do you store stress?" Members then organize themselves in a line according to where they store it, beginning with those who feel stress in the head area and ending at the feet. Form a circle staying in the same order. Starting from the top (the head or neck), each person demonstrates an exercise that s/he does to relax that part of the body. Everyone then tries out the motion. This process continues around the circle until each person has had a turn. This is very effective when done non-verbally.

Dance Cards
One card is passed out to each group member. On each card is an image of a person, animal or object. The leader starts the music and invites participants to interpret the image using some movement. Group members exchange cards as part of the activity.

Sound and Motion Pass
Group members form a circle allowing distance between themselves for movement. One participant (the "leader") creates a motion and sound and "passes" them to the person on his/her right. The motion and sound are then imitated by this person and passed on, until they return to the original leader. A second leader then chooses a motion and sound and the process is repeated.

Hand-On-Hand
Two partners face one another and decide on who is "leader" and who is "follower." The leader's hands are upturned; the follower's hands are placed, turned downward, on top of the leader's. The leader moves his/her hands in any direction in a gentle rhythm and the follower responds accordingly. This activity is similar to "Mirroring" except physical touch is included.

Scarf Dance
The group forms a circle. Each participant holds colored fabric, ribbon or crepe paper in each hand. Each person in turn uses the strips to make a movement such as arm circling, jumping over strips or twirling. As each person shows his/her version of the dance, everyone else imitates the movement.

Walking/Moving with Partner
The group is divided into partners. One person (A) leads the other person (B) around the room. At first (B) is passive and trusting and moves as directed. Then (B) begins to offer some resistance. Finally (B) very actively resists (A's) attempts at moving him/her. Reverse roles and then discuss what occurred.

Movement Through
Using your imagination, move through:

- honey
- sand
- daisies in a field
- jungle underbrush
- a large bubble gum bubble
- water
- air
- lime Jell-O
- clouds
- a deep pocket full of odds and ends

Eye Contact
Standing or sitting in a circle, each participant tries to make eye contact with another person. When the contact has been acknowledged by a given signal (pointing or a nod of the head, for in-

stance), the two switch places as quickly as possible. This exercise facilitates eye contact with little threat (in the context of the game), and helps increase observational skills.

Exploration of Trust and Support

Group members stand in large circle holding hands. They pull away from each other while maintaining balance; they lean in; lean to the right and to the left; lean on one another.

Alphabet Movement

Moving through the alphabet from A to Z — using animals or object names that start with each consecutive letter, a dance or movement is made up for each. For example, "Move like an 'A'...alligator, 'B'...ball, 'C'...caterpillar." Encourage dancers to call out suggestions for each letter.

The "Land of S" Action Verbs

Group members move to the "S" action verbs, e.g.: sliding, skipping, slumping, sauntering, strolling, striking, strutting, stomping, slithering, snapping, smashing. Leader or group members can call out suggestions.

Moving to Opposites

These activities help group members explore ways of moving and the use of space. The leader can ask for movement suggestions from the group.

- Open-closed
- High-low
- Large-small
- Heavy-light
- Near-far
- Wide-narrow
- Straight-slanted
- Linear-curved

Footprints

The leader creates footprints out of heavy, colored paper or vinyl and creates a pattern for the dancers to follow. (Make sure that the clients don't slip — tape the footprints onto the floor well!)

Moving to Divergent Emotions

Exploring these contradictory emotions will produce a wide range of movements. The leader can ask for suggestions from the group to build a longer list of emotional opposites.

- Love — hate
- Lost — found
- Knowledge — ignorance
- Happy — sad

Complementary Stretching

In pairs, dancers engage in various exercises using each other's weight, strength and balance to stretch.

Mirroring in Groups of Four

Mirroring may begin with partners taking turns being leader or follower, then reversing roles. Pairs then move into groups of four. In these groups, one member is the leader and three are following. The leader's goal now is to pick up on movements made by the other three members of the group. Can group members find a balance between who is "leading" and who is "following?"

Create a Dance

In groups of four, participants create a dance (given about 5 minutes to make it up) and then perform it for the entire group.

Contact Improvisation

Pairs explore movement together — a good activity for "staying in the moment." The group divides into partners. Pairs are then given the following instructions: Keep your eyes open, be alert; look for opportunities to support your partner (e.g., move in underneath them), but don't give or take weight without listening for/feeling the agreement of your partner's body. Let each movement evolve from mutual agreement rather than letting an image in your own mind dictate what happens next. Mutual trust is based on "uncompromising attention." *(Exposed To Gravity Project)*

Circle Walk

The group forms a large circle. Begin the activity by facing forward with left sides toward center of the circle. Count together and walk, one step to each count; 1, 2, 3, 4, 5, 6, 7, 8, 9, 10, 11, 12, 13, 14, 15, 16. On the count of 16 turn to face the opposite direction and count and step 1-15. You have subtracted one step. On the count of 15 turn again and count and step 1-14. Continue to the end of counting.

You Can Tell How I Feel by the Way that I _____

Group members takes turns using their creativity to express emotions through movement and/or facial expressions. Each person demonstrates how s/he feels while the other members look on. The leader can ask for more suggestions for expression.

- walk
- hop
- wiggle
- scream
- skip
- smile
- stomp
- spin

Example: You can tell how I feel by the way that I...walk

This chant is one that either the group or the dancer can do while s/he demonstrates in movement how s/he feels:

the way that I ...(walk)
the way that I...(walk)
You can tell how I feel by the way that I ...(walk)
walk
walk
walk

Think of Someone Who Moves the Way You'd Like To...

Group members imitate the style of someone they admire. Each individual performs (e.g., a walk, gestures, body language) while others in the group observe.

Letting Go and Holding On

Group members are asked to react physically to the question: "How would you look if you were letting go of _____ and moving towards _____."

Example:
"How would you look if you were letting go of *fear* (hunching shoulders, hands in front of face) and moving towards *trust* (standing straight, opening up)?"
Other possibilities: anger, sadness, pain.

Suggesting Movements and Varying Them

The leader suggests a series of movements for group members to make and then varies them — a spatial exploration exercise. The leader might, for example, suggest making a pantomime movement of painting a fence. S/he could then call out suggestions for modifying the painting motion: faster, slower, smaller, larger, higher, lower, rougher, smoother.

Closure

Each member of the group creates and uses a gesture (small movement, e.g., tipping hat) as their personal sign off at the end of a session.

Movement Map

Each member of the group draws a map of his/her movement path. For example, the map may show "3 hops, 4 slides and a turn, then change directions, and so on." S/he dances it, then finds a partner and they guide one other through their maps.

Body Talk

Every participant makes two cards — one with a single emotion and another card with a single body part. The emotions cards are put into one hat and the body parts are put into another. Participants take turns drawing a card from each hat (one emotion, one body part). Using only the body part indicated on the card, the participant displays the emotion found on the second card. The rest of the participants guess the emotion and body part.

Elbow Tag

The leader divides the group into sets of three. The "center" person links elbows with the two on either side of him/her. One group is designated "it." One person in the "it" group receives a "marker," such as a scarf. This threesome then separates to act as three separate individuals.

Action: The person with the marker tries to tag either of the two free runners from his/her group. These two runners each try to join elbows with some other threesome. When a threesome becomes a foursome, the fourth person (the person on the opposite end from the former free runner) becomes "it." The threesomes move as units around the area trying to avoid free runners.

Object: Try not to become "it."

Back to Back

The leader divides the group into pairs. Each pair first sits on the ground, back to back. Participants then bend their knees, pulling them up to their chests, keeping their feet on the ground. The leader instructs each pair to hook their elbows together. Working together and using the combined strength of their backs, each pair tries to "stand up" together simultaneously. This may be a new and difficult experience for some participants. Also, having slippery socks (no shoes) or slippery floor might create an added difficulty. The leader stresses working together and using combined strength — then the task can be done fairly easily.

Writing Your Name with an Imaginary Pen

The leader suggests a part of the body, then asks the participant to pretend to hold an imaginary pen with that body part and to write his/her name using as much space as necessary. For example, the leader might say, "Write your name using your head."

Movement Exploration

Movement exploration, long an accepted part of elementary education, is a set of progressive problem solving experiences designed to teach a person to control body movements and improve physical skills. (Deighton, 1971). The basis of movement exploration lies in exploring fundamental patterns of physical activity — both locomotor (e.g., running, skipping, walking) and non-locomotor (e.g., bending, pushing, pulling). This exploration is important to children and adults, but especially important in improving the physical and perceptual abilities of people with disabilities.

Educational Goals

These goals might be taught as "learning units," in the following progression:

Safety
This should be the first item covered in a lesson or set of activities. When a whistle is blown, participants must learn to stop, look and listen.

Body Image and Spatial Awareness
A very important aspect of movement exploration is learning about the body: What are the parts of the body, how do they move and in how many different ways? How can they be used in skilled activities and how can they be used in combinations with other body parts? How does your body fit into the environment around it and how do you move through the environment avoiding obstacles and maneuvering safely?

Self-Confidence, Self-Assurance and Solving Challenges
The challenges in question may include going to greater heights, maneuvering over a narrow surface or a broad expanse, covering unstable ground, or even traveling safely at high speed. The theory

is that people will have a tendency to take their success in meeting challenges and generalize it to other activities.

Visual Focus and Balance

These two abilities are considered together because of the influence of balance on focus. Balance is, in and of itself, fundamental to almost all motor tasks: sitting, kneeling, standing, walking — even sleeping on one side. Most learning tasks require visual focus, the ability to focus on a something and maintain the connection. If balance is poor, a person's field of vision may shift frequently in the attempt to maintain some kind of balance.

Strength and Endurance

Both strength and endurance are basic to successful movement, health and safety. For example: strength is needed to pull yourself to safety from a dangerous situation, while endurance is critical to performing throughout an active day, with energy to spare for engaging in special play time after work or in case of emergency.

Hand-Eye Coordination

Use of hand-eye coordination enables a person to be a part of the action in games, especially ball games. Hand-eye coordination is also important in reading, writing and most creative endeavors.

Movement Exploration Activities

Each activity in this series is formulated as a set of directions which can be given to a group by a leader or therapist:

Individual Activities

Body Parts to the Floor
Find a way to touch different numbers of body parts to the floor. (The leader calls out how many: 4, 3, 2, 1, etc.)

Finding a Space

- Find a place in the room — a place you feel drawn to
    - Find three points of the space that will help you "find your way home" to that place (e.g., to a mark on the floor or wall)
    - Pretend you have a paint brush and decorate your space

- Begin to move through your space.
    - How slowly can you move?
    - How gently? softly?
    - How low can you move?
    - How high can you move?
    - Can you find a middle height to move with?

- How can you form the first letter of your name while staying in your space?
    - Print your first name within your space.
    - Can you use the top half of your body to form your name?
    - Can you use the lower part?
    - Can you write your name using your whole body?

- Leave your "home base" and begin to meet your neighbors and see your neighborhood.

Walking the Line

Walk a line on the floor (the leader can make a line with masking tape or use a pattern in the floor).

More Movement Practice

Move as if you are moving through space now — without music. How small can you be? (Make a sound that goes with it, if you can). How light and feathery can you be? How proud? How large? Do a silly walk. Walk as if you are very heavy, as if on a planet where you weigh more than you do on earth. Feel the weight of your steps.

Pair Activities

Body Parts Game
Call out two body parts. Group members find a partner and touch these two parts together (e.g., one partner's nose to the other's elbow). Participants are asked to find a new partner for each new challenge. Examples:

- nose to elbow
- knee to elbow
- shoulder to shoulder
- hand to back
- hand to foot
- chin to ear

If possible, ask group members to call out two (appropriate) body parts.

Pattern Walk
Using a large piece of paper and a crayon, each person draws a pattern, walks it and then leads his/her partner through the pattern. The pattern can, for example, consist of varying step sizes, turns, twist, circles and gaps.

Bubbles
Remind the group of what happens when a bubble comes in contact with other bubbles — they can become a bubble cluster! With your partner begin moving around the room, bumping into other pairs to become groups of: 4, 8, 16.

Mirroring Movement
Find a partner and mirror each other's moves. See how many ways you can challenge yourselves with tests of your balance and visual focus.

Group Activities

"Touch Blue" Game

Start the game by reminding everyone to be gentle and appropriate in their touching. One person is designated as "it." Ask everyone except "it" to get into the position of "touch blue" (touch someone who is wearing blue). The "it" person calls out a series of other colors ("touch red," "touch black") for participants to locate and touch. At some point, the person who is "it" calls "touch blue" and everyone must rush to find blue before "it" tags him/her. The one who is tagged becomes "it."

Animal House

This activity will use total imagination. First set the scene:
- Ask everyone to think of an animal that they wish to be for this session and how they might imitate this animal's movements.
- Encourage the group to use facial expressions, to walk, crawl and/or make sounds to show what animals they "are."
- Tell the group that the theme will be set in the jungle.

Then set everything in motion by speaking to the group and giving them the following instructions: "As the group moves around on the mats, each of you will encounter other creatures and must decide what you will do as you approach other animals. Will you run, or snarl or just look curious? Will you fly away or swim? How do you react to being in the jungle? Are you scared or do you rule the jungle? Are you large or small? Two-legged or four? Are you loud or quiet? Continue moving among the group until you have found a position among the rest of the group that shows what animal you are and who you might 'hang out with.'"

Animals

1. The group forms a circle.
2. Each member chooses a favorite animal s/he wishes to act out.

3. The leader begins by imitating his/her favorite animal. S/he travels towards any person in the group and greets that person as his/her animal would greet any other animal.
4. The person being greeted should respond in her animal character and then approach another member in the group.
5. Continue until all members have had a chance to demonstrate an animal.

The Human See-Saw
1. Divide into two groups and form two lines facing one another.
2. Group One goes from a standing position to the floor in a way specified by the leader (e.g., quickly, slowly, like a cat).
3. Then Group One watches as Group Two moves from the floor to a standing position (the reverse of Group One) in some specified way.
4. The groups continue to take turns, moving up and down like a see-saw. At some point they switch (Group Two starting first from a standing position).
5. This up and down activity may continue until all ways have been explored.

The ways of getting up and down may be designated by the leader or group members may make suggestions. Each group may also be given a list of ways to get up and down and may choose from the list.

Ways to go down:
- in awe or worship
- formally and gracefully
- as a melting snowman (or woman — would she melt differently?)
- slipping on something slick
- after losing a long distance race
- after winning a long distance race
- to tie a child's shoelace

Ways to get up:
- waking up after sleeping on the floor
- someone you love has come into the room
- like a child who is caught somewhere s/he's not supposed to be
- you heard a loud crash outside
- you smell smoke
- a dancer on stage

Activities Using Equipment

Ball Movement Activities
- Show how quietly you can come up, get a ball and, without touching each other, go back to your space.
- How many body parts can you bounce the ball with?
  - How many times can you bounce the ball in one minute?
  - How many times can you throw the ball up and catch it in one minute?
- Choose a partner — you should each have a ball. Toss one of the balls back and forth; start close and slowly increase the distance.
  - How many ways can you throw the ball to each other?
  - Introduce the second ball and find way(s) to keep the balls moving in opposite directions.
- How quickly can you can return the balls without touching each other?

Hula Hoop Activities
Individual Activities
- Show how tall you can be as you come up to get your hula hoop. Holding your hoop, how high can you stretch?
- Can you hold a hoop above your head and drop it so that it hits the ground without touching your body?
- Can you spin a hoop and keep it going like an egg beater?

- Can you jump in and out of the hoop while holding on to one part?
- Being careful not to bump into anyone, can you roll your hoop in a straight line and keep it from falling over?
- Can you change direction? Right? Left?
- How fast can you roll your hoop?
- How slowly can you roll your hoop?
- Can you roll your hoop on the floor so that it will roll back to you?

Pair Activities
- Can you exchange hoops with a partner by rolling them back and forth?
- Can you create a rhythm? How fast? How slow?
- Who can jump into a hoop held by your partner? Now, let your partner try.
- Your partner is going to hold two hoops in different positions. Can you go through both hoops? Let your partner try.
- Can you and your partner exchange hoops by throwing and catching them at the same time? Can you catch a hoop which has been thrown by your partner, on your arm?

Musical Hoops — Non-Eliminative
Hoops are laid on the floor — at first there is one for everyone. The game begins with each person standing in his/her own hoop. The music starts, everyone steps out of the hoop and one or two hoops are removed by the leader. Everyone begins moving through the hoops. When the music stops, everyone must stand inside a hoop. Some people will end up sharing a hoop. The elimination of hoops continues in each round, and each time more people have to double or triple up inside the hoops. Finally at the end the entire group is squeezed into one or two hoops. There is a lot of physical contact and laughter.

Creating Obstacle Courses

Divide people into groups of three or four. Each group creates an obstacle course using the hula hoops and themselves as challenges to be gotten around. Then take turns trying out each other's creations.

Collecting the Hoops

1. Line up. Each person gets a hoop and puts it on his/her right arm.
2. Everybody then puts his/her left arm through someone else's hoop and holds hands, until everyone is joined together in a circle, with hands joined and each hoop between two people and over their arms.
3. One person is the end of the line; his/her right hand is not joined.
4. S/he will get "buried" by all the hoops. Starting to the right, the hoops are transferred by each person all the way around the circle, over people's bodies until they all get to him/her.
5. This is done with everyone *holding hands* with the person next to him/her.

Parachute Activities

Roll the parachute inward to form a sturdy handle.

- How far back can you stand, still holding the parachute?
- How far overhead can you stretch? How low to the ground?
- How can we make waves using the parachute?
- Can you run in a circle holding the parachute extended overhead with the right hand?
- Show how you would raise the chute overhead, then release it and re-grasp it while it is floating in space.

Dance Therapy Resources

Organizations

American Dance Therapy Association (ADTA)
2000 Century Plaza, Suite 108
Columbia, MD 21044
phone: 410-997-4040
fax: 410-997-4048

Northern California Chapter of the ADTA
Carrie Queene, Newsletter Editor
433 Haddon
Oakland, CA 94606
phone: 510-893-4669

Books

Chace, M., S. Chaiklin, S. Sandel, and A. Ohn (ed.). 1993. **Foundations of Dance/Movement Therapy: The Life and Work of Marian Chace.** Columbia, MD: American Dance Therapy Association.

Chaiklin, H., ed. 1975. **Marian Chace: Her Papers**. Columbia, MD: American Dance Therapy Association.

Levy, F. J. 1995. **Dance and Other Expressive Art Therapies**. New York, NY: Routledge.

Zwerling, I. 1979. "The Creative Art Therapies as 'Real Therapies.' " *Journal of Hospital and Community Psychiatry.* 30(12).

14

Poetry and Writing

The experience of writing is an introspective and personal process. Individuals who write poetry or keep a journal will attest to the power of writing down thoughts and feelings on paper. The very process of writing may lead a writer to discoveries about him/herself that lie hidden from conscious thought. Creative writing is a powerful tool for examining and/or exposing personal feelings, attitudes and beliefs. In creative writing, ideas emerge from our life history, culture and times, as well as our heart, intellect and spirit. In writing creatively, an individual makes the statement, "This is me, this is what I believe, see, feel and think about."

For some people, writing is a haven where they can freely express whatever they choose to say, and be assured of at least one avid reader...themselves. Others, who have a heroic struggle putting their thoughts on paper, may perceive writing as a chore. As therapists interested in developing a creative writing group, we need to examine our own feelings about writing before we can guide others.

Why Use Creative Writing as Therapy?

Some of the reasons include:
- Sharing with others establishes a sense of community.
- Sometimes writing may be easier than speaking.
- Sometimes we can learn about ourselves.
- Sometimes we can learn about others.
- Writing spontaneously can be a gift from our unconscious.
- Sharing our writing can invite others to look through our eyes.

Why Use Poetry Therapy?

Poetry therapy is based on the principle that by writing poetry, reading it, or both, the individual will be encouraged to express his/her thoughts and find greater awareness and self-understanding.

In **Poetry Therapy** edited by Dr. Jack Leedy (1969), the purpose of poetry therapy is twofold:
- By writing verse, the individual is encouraged to voice fears, doubts and anxieties that s/he might otherwise not share with others. The individual may also be able to use writing as a source of emotional release (e.g., if you can't say it, write it).
- By reading poetry others have written, an individual may find:
  - someone with whom to identify.
  - a springboard for discussion.
  - the opportunity to share with others.

Guidelines for the Creative Writing Group

Objectives
- to offer comfort or support
- to increase insight into self or others
- to increase empathy

- to foster creative growth
- to encourage imagination
- to build self-confidence in writing abilities
- to increase socialization skills
- to amuse

How to Give People Permission to Write (Unlock the Blocks)

Let participants know the following:
- Anything they have written is acceptable.
- The focus of the group is on creative expression only.
- No one will care about spelling, grammar, punctuation or handwriting.
- There will be no red pencils or grades.
- Sharing is optional.
- The group is only interested in your ideas, not in analyzing your creation. Analysis is only important in terms of what the writer does with his/her own work.

Thoughts for the Therapist

- What is the goal of this writing group? What is the purpose of writing?
- People are like crystals — with a full range of personalities. Different aspects of people may emerge from their writing.
- Don't be afraid that no one will write.
- If you as the therapist say everything is acceptable/okay, you need to really believe that.
- Writing can give a vision concrete power.
- Honor each person's work/effort.
- Don't deny anything that is going on, whether it is a new idea or an interpersonal development.

- Be mindful not to set a standard, so that group members are not tempted to compare themselves.
- Try it yourself first. Test a writing activity to see how it works and how long it takes to do it.
- Keep your own journal of thoughts, poetry and ideas so that you are as involved in the writing process as your clients are.

Different Levels of Meaning

People may respond:
- As they really are.
- As they would like to be.
- With whatever pops into their minds.

Group Process

- **Warm-up.** This is optional. As with other creative arts groups, a warm-up activity helps focus the group before doing the main activity.
- **Introducing the activity.** Be able to give the group an accurate idea of what to expect and how long the activity will take (familiarize yourself with it beforehand).
- **Doing the activity.** Allow enough time — everyone thinks and writes at a different rate.
- **Closing.** Provide time for sharing a gentle closing, feedback and validation.

Different Kinds of Groups

Writing groups takes shape for a variety of reasons. Creative writing groups or poetry groups are organized to develop writing skills related to poetry, short stories or any kind of narrative writing. They can also be used as a therapeutic arts group. Some groups get together to produce a newspaper/newsletter to publicize information about the facility, participants or upcoming events. Other groups, especially in long term care settings, get together for purposes of compiling life histories/reviews — for reminiscing. Bifolkal is an organization that deals with the issue of creating oral histories. Other writing can be done on an individual basis, such as: journal writing, diary and letter writing.

Different Kinds of Writing

Different kinds of writing are adaptable to different group purposes. No matter what the purpose, all styles used for therapeutic reasons fall into a class of writing called the "Personal-Emotive," which is employed to express personal thoughts and feelings. Listed below are some of the specific types of writing adaptable for therapeutic purposes. Warm-up exercises and two writing activities that are particularly well-suited to groups are then considered in detail.

Reasons for Writing

- **For venting.** Graffiti or a private diary/journal — helps the writer to think, reflect, stay in touch with self. Written from the heart, it may be cathartic. Not meant to be read by others. No editing, just immediate reactions (and possibly fresh insights) regarding daily events.
- **For reflection and/or sharing.** May be autobiographical, reminiscing, life history, oral history. Increases self-esteem — goals may be socialization. Example: group newspaper.
- **For fun.** Humorous narratives, short stories, descriptive pieces.
- **For imagination.** Writing about utopia, a projection of the future, the self in a different setting, alternate worlds or other people.
- **For poetic expression.** Haiku, free verse, sonnets or simple rhymes — all can carry the feelings and emotions of the writer.

Warm-up Exercises

Even experienced writers need to warm-up/prepare for writing. These exercises focus the mind and/or produce ideas that can be used in the main activity. These warm-ups also eliminate the fear of the blank piece of paper — once they're done, the page is no longer empty and the individual has begun writing. One excellent exercise is *free writing.* In this technique, the person is instructed to write a stream of consciousness (whatever comes to mind) for a limited period of time. Some writers start every day with 10 minutes of free writing to clear their mind of all the things which distract them, "to give the barking dog a bone," as one writer once put it. Another excellent warm-up comes from a book by Gabriele Rico (1983) called **Writing the Natural Way** and it is called *clustering.* In this technique, one word acts as the stimulus for recording all the associations that spring to mind in a brief period of time. This is further described in the Poetry and Writing Activities section found further on in this chapter.

Themes

Holidays, seasons, pets or life issues (e.g., birth or death) are examples of themes that can be very effective as the basis for writing. Use the senses to engage memory and begin the writing process. If the topic is "summer," for instance, bring in seashells, tanning lotion, or sand — anything that evokes the "essence" of summer. Ask the group to suggest other things that symbolize summer. These suggestions could be the basis for individual poems or even a group poem such as a *renga* (everyone writes one line, word or phrase on an agreed upon theme). Contributions to the renga may be public (e.g., stating them out loud to the group) or private (e.g., each person writes a line without seeing the other lines). Often, in the private method, the other lines are masked from each writer until the whole piece is revealed by the leader who reads all the lines together. The lines always seem to come together as a whole.

Poetry Readings

Reading poetry inspires writers of poetry. Having group members recite and listen to poetry will help them learn new language and ways of expressing ideas and sensitize them to the rhythms of poetry. In conducting poetry readings, remember to:

- Choose poems with understandable language.
- Choose poems that represent a variety of emotions and experiences.
- Provide each person with a copy of the poem, if possible or appropriate (and if permissible, given copyright laws).
- Ask how the group responded to the poem: feelings, opinions.
- Bring poetry books and ask participants to find a favorite one to share.
- Tape or record the poetry reading and then play it back for people to hear.
- Ask for someone whose native language is not English to read a poem in his/her native language and to translate it.

Ideas for Writing

Ideas for writing can come from almost anywhere. The following is a summary of some of the ways to stimulate group writing.

Word Associations

Stereotypes

- women
- men
- ethnic groups
- mountain folk
- bigots

Themes

- holidays
- life issues

Free Association

- summer
- men
- women
- happiness
- hope
- ambition
- life
- love
- pain
- death
- I am

Writing in Response

— to a story, poem, statement, song, picture, etc.

Forms of Writing

Poetry (a few examples)

- free verse
- sonnet
- renga, haiku, syntu
- limericks
- diamonte

Autobiographical

- life histories
- oral histories
- reminiscing
- life review

Letter Writing

- to others
- to self

Newspaper/Newsletter

- about the facility, its participants or events

Personal Reflection

- sharing of wisdom
- journal
- epitaph

Projection and Association

- statement completion
- clustering

Writing Games

Games that help individuals sharpen creative thinking and word skills include: *Shufflebook*, *Mad Libs* and *Flabbergast*. These are available in toy and specialty stores. Crossword puzzles and other word games may also help in developing writing and thinking skills. Advanced groups can try creating their own crossword puzzles.

Eleven Writing Exercises

The exercises listed below are for the most part short and to the point. There may be a therapeutic aspect to their content, but as a rule they are less psychologically intense than the guided activities which appear in the following section. They are the written equivalent of theater games, meant to foster spontaneity and creative thinking.

- Title Creation:
  Write a title for the following types of writing:
  - a detective novel
  - love poems
  - a science fiction story
  - a romance novel
  - a great adventure
  - a gothic horror story
- Write your own epitaph.
- Spell names backwards (moorssalc = classroom).
- Create a poem or short story; each person adds a line or a paragraph.
- Write a situation from another person's point of view.
- Write a letter to: mother, father, old friend, former teacher, former lover, President, spiritual guide, higher self, someone you resent in regards to "unresolved business."
- You are given $500,000 tax free: What would you do?
- The medicine person of a tribe wants to talk to the children about adulthood and growing up: What does s/he want them to know? Parenting? Work? Love? Courage? Fun?
- Make up a dream or fantasy life and write as if you were someone else.
- Design a perfect resort for yourself. Where would it be? What could you do there?
- Recall an embarrassing moment (e.g., getting a traffic ticket). What were you thinking of at the time?

This next set of exercises are formally named, but are still basically simple exercises.

Personal Associations/Extensions of Self
Provide a list of ideas or ask participants to come up with their own. What would I be like if I were a:

- book
- type of weather
- piece of clothing
- period in time
- dance
- song

Images of Self
- Are there any images of yourself that get you in trouble sometimes?
- Are there healthy ones you want to retain?
- Is there something from your pocket or purse, or something you are wearing that has meaning for you?

Props — To Evoke Characters
We all have met interesting characters in our lives. The introduction of props can jog memories of people we have known or seen. Ask questions such as these about each piece of clothing: Who wore this? Who would wear this?

- Hats
- Shoes
- Jewelry
- Purses
- T-shirt

Three Wishes
You will be granted three wishes; erase one, then erase another. Which wish remains? Which ones did you let go?

Dialogue
Write a dialogue between a person (mother, friend, family, boss, spiritual guide, self) and a *drug* (your favorite drug or food that is most difficult to refuse/limit).

Three Envelopes
Three envelopes are filled with slips of paper by the leader. Each one deals with a different type of subject and contains:
1. names of things (work, walkie-talkie)
2. names of people/occupations, etc. (story character, a 90 year old grandfather, female astronaut)
3. names of places/or events (marriage, birthday)

Choose one slip of paper from each of the three envelopes and make up a paragraph incorporating the things, people and places.

Visualization Journal
Use the script in Chapter 15 (*Meditation and Creative Visualization*) called "Advisor." Do the visualization and then write about the gift or advice received from your Spiritual Guide. Writing about the visualization solidifies the experience, bringing insight and comfort. It can be a good, healing exercise.

Poetry and Writing Activities

The following activities are described in the context of particular therapeutic goals that the therapist may have for the group.

Back Drawing and Writing
Goals: A good warm-up activity; introductory contact between participants.
Description: The leader divides the group into pairs. One of the partners sits and becomes a "canvas" while the other partner is the "artist." Using one finger, the standing "artist" draws a shape or a figure on the seated person's back. Seated person reproduces that form on a piece of paper. Then together, the partners write what comes to mind about the symbol and the experience.
Materials: Pen/pencil, paper.
Setting: Chairs (for "canvases" to sit on) generously spaced around a table. The leader demonstrates and explains that the artist

should draw slowly so that the "canvas" can understand what is being drawn.

Zen Telegram and Planting Ceremony

Goals: This is a non-threatening activity. Participants work individually as well as together. May be used as an introduction to creative expression.

Description: The group close their eyes and are encouraged to get into a meditative mood. They then make any marking (e.g., symbol, geometric figure, random mark) they care to make on their paper. When they are satisfied that they are finished, participants open their eyes and write any word or phrase on the paper which the marking brings to mind. Discussion follows for those who wish to comment on their reaction to the exercise.

Adaptations: A follow-up activity is to mark the paper in the same manner (but not the same configuration), as in the first activity. When eyes are opened, all participants pass their "telegrams" on to the person sitting next to them, who then writes any word or phrase which comes to mind about the mark on the paper. Discussion follows.

Materials: Tape or CD player, Japanese tapes or CDs, small plant pots, soil, water source and seedlings, Japanese paint brushes, India ink or paint, newsprint paper.

Setting: Soothing Japanese music is playing as the session starts. Facilitator welcomes everyone, discusses intent of program, and talks about creative growth. A planting ceremony takes place in which each participant plants a seedling in a pot as a symbol of the expected growth of everyone in the group, singly and together, in the coming weeks.

You'll Never Believe...

Description: This is an exercise in guided creative writing. The facilitator establishes the parameters of the writing by using a phrase as the format and defining the elements for the clients to include in writing. For example:

1. "You'll never believe who I saw!" — Name one person, one word that describes a person, and one place. The participant could write, "I saw kind Whoopi Goldberg in the kitchen."
2. "You'll never believe what I ate." — Name one food, one word for flavor, and one place. "I ate a sweet strawberry in the back yard." Participants may read their sentences aloud.

Adaptations: In the beginning, the number of elements can be varied (e.g., just name a person) depending on the abilities of the group. Add more elements as the group proceeds through the activity.

Materials: Pen/pencil and paper.

Group size: Do not make the group too large — a smaller writing group allows the facilitator to give proper attention to each client.

Pictures and Words

Description: Pick a painting that lends itself to story telling. Put someone in charge of writing down what is said about the painting by the group members. Let your imagination fly. Expand what you see. Example: *Girl, girl crying, girl sitting.*

Now expand the story by asking questions, "Why is she sitting?" *Girl crying, waiting for her mother to come home.*

Finish the project when the time period or story ideas end. Read what was written, as is. For a cohesive finale, hang the picture and story in a common space so all clients can enjoy their project.

Adaptations: Anything that is said about a picture can be written down by the leader; clients can draw, and the leader can write a story about each person's drawing. Sharing the story may be a teaching method to get individuals interested in telling stories about themselves.

Materials: Any painting that lends itself to storytelling.

Group Size: Any, but a group numbering over 25 may need to be split up into smaller groups.

Statement Completion
Directions: Write down the following partial statements and complete them:
- It makes me mad when …
- I suppose…
- I have…
- Don't you hate it when…
- Just when…
- I need…
- When I get mad I…

Adaptations: If the participants are unable to write, the facilitator may write for them. If a participant cannot think of a completion to a statement, move on to another statement. Similarly if the participant can't think of a response to a word, or any other ways to complete the sentence, move on.
Materials: Pen/pencil, paper.
Group Size: 2 or more.

Word Response
Directions: The leader reads off each word, allowing time for participants to write down the word(s) which each subject brings to mind.
- Men
- Women
- Summer
- Pain
- Happiness
- Death
- Hope
- Ambition
- Life
- Love

Adaptations: See *Statement Completion* above.
Materials: Pen/pencil, paper.
Group Size: 2 or more.

I Am
Directions: Leader instructs participants to write down the phrase "I am...," and complete it as many ways as they would like to. For example:
- I am...lovable
- I am...blue-eyed.
- I am...lazy.

Adaptations: See *Statement Completion* above.
Materials: Pen/pencil, paper.
Group Size: 2 or more.

Small Potato Touch
Goals: To facilitate small group cooperation and to foster using senses other than sight, to introduce the senses as a creative medium.
Description: The group is divided into smaller groups which are given a bag apiece. Each bag contains one item — perhaps a piece of rope, a silver dollar, or a dried herb — and, without looking at the item, each person in the group feels it, smells it and passes it on to the others. When all have examined it thoroughly it is returned to the bag and the group members open their eyes. Each person takes a strip of paper, writes a line about the item, and tapes it onto the full sheet of paper provided. The group may arrange the order of statements to create the group poem. Each completed sheet of paper is hung on the wall, and the collective group discusses its reactions to the activity. The group may wish to guess what was in each bag which did not belong to them by the evidence written on the strips.
Materials: A number of miscellaneous items of widely varying properties of smell and touch, and paper bags for each item. Scotch tape, paper in strips, full sheets of paper.
Setting: Group sits at five separate tables of five chairs each. Facilitator reads the poem, "The Blind Men and the Elephant," which addresses the idea of identifying an object without the sense of vision.

Our Memory Poem

Goals: To facilitate large group participation and cooperation to explore the creation of poetry. To increase awareness through visual stimulation.

Description: Each person writes one line or image that describes a childhood memory. The facilitator collects the lines from each person and randomly places them on a large table or on a bulletin board. Working together the group decides the order of the lines and arranges them. The group then picks a title for its poem. Another possibility is that the facilitator puts the lines in order and the group creates the title or titles for the work.

Materials: Use whatever helps create a mood from the past. Items could include an old table cloth, magazines, old toys, clothes, photographs. A tape recorder could play old music. Pieces of paper and pens for individual writing. A place to combine paper — e.g., newsprint, a bulletin board, table.

Setting: Each old item may be discussed by the group or participants may look at items as they wish. The facilitator may read nursery rhymes or other poems by Robert Louis Stevenson, Gabriela Mistral, Langston Hughes and others that evoke childhood.

Resources:
- "Some Good Things to Be Said for the Iron Age" by Gary Snyder
- "The Language" by Robert Creeley
- "This is Just to Say" by William Carlos Williams
- "Snow" by Lovis NocNeile
- "The Blessing" by James Wright

Holiday Memories

Goals: To share the holiday, recall previous happy holidays, feel connected to the holiday and each other. To stimulate creativity through the senses of taste and smell.

Description: Participants are asked to pick out the most memorable Thanksgiving they can recall, and in a half an hour or less to write about it. Participants are then encouraged to share what has been written with the group. Writing may be in prose or poetry, and it is stressed that principles of detail are equally applicable to prose or poetry.

Materials: Pens, paper.

Setting: If possible, pie (preferably fresh baked) and coffee are waiting in a nearby kitchen to be served during the discussion. The group talks about what Thanksgiving means to them and the pros and cons of holidays in general.

Resources:

- "The First Thanksgiving" by Jennifer Mulondy
- "In Appreciation" by John Silver

Clustering/Wandering with Words

Goals: To teach a brainstorming technique. To let participant be involved in a creative experience that can bring insight.

Description: The leader suggests a word for the nucleus of the cluster, or each participant picks a word that holds emotional content for him/her. It could be someone's name, a place, a color, food, smell, year, etc. Be sure it's just one word. That word is written down and circled. The participants let their thoughts wander, allowing any connections to the word to come into their heads. Write these down quickly, each in its own circle, in a line from the nucleus word. As the associations grow, some words that arise may relate directly to the nucleus word; others may relate to an associated word. Connect words with lines to the appropriate association.

Materials: Pens, paper and music.

Setting: Facilitator begins by asking participants to share one word. Then questions may be asked to help stimulate "word wandering" such as, "How does your word feel? How does it smell? Is it strong?" Another technique is to simply play music and allow participants to take their time and wander as they wish.

Toy Talk

Goals: To encourage reminiscence. To engage in a guided fantasy experience.

Description: This is a creative writing exercise based on fantasy. Participants select two toys from those placed in front of the group. Participants become acquainted with their choices, make up names for them, decide where the toys come from and if they (the toys) have a message for participants. Participants write a paragraph describing a conversation the two toys would have or some experience the toys shared.

Materials: Pens/pencils/crayons, paper, a variety of small toys (e.g., dolls, balls, trucks).

Setting: If working with young adults or adults, the leader may need to reconnect the group to childhood and the roles that toys played in their lives. Possibly use creative visualization to take the group back to childhood and "their favorite toys."

I Remember

Goals: To formulate and express appreciation of another person.

Description: This exercise can be done in more than one way. Participants can create their own entire poem, or contribute words or lines. The idea is to write a poem honoring someone who has left the group. For this purpose, a poem will be described as: "The simple, clear expression of a fully felt experience."

1. In writing the poem — I remember ... (person's name).
2. Describe the person's appearance or demeanor (flowing hair, twinkling eyes, raucous laugh).
3. Describe some quality, value or attitude of the person (their generosity, willingness to fight, shyness).
4. Describe an experience shared with the person (a conversation, a walk, studying together, riding home, time in class).
5. If possible, summarize with a description of feeling about the person. (This is not always necessary).

Materials: Pens/pencils, paper.

Setting: The leader may want to start this activity by initiating a brief reminiscence about a person who has left the group, in order to bring this individual into the group's consciousness.

Writing Gifts

Goals: Gain experience in giving and receiving gifts/thoughts; social skills development.

Description: Each person selects a subject on which s/he wishes to receive a thought, a sort of "gift" in writing. For example, if the subject is peace, the thought may be, "have peaceful interactions with family members." Requests are written on pieces of paper, collected and handed out to other group members randomly. Each group member writes a thought on the paper s/he receives and returns it to the original person. The recipient reads their gift aloud.

Variation: One participant makes a request for thoughts to the entire group and the other group members respond.

Materials: Colored pens/pencils, paper.

Setting: The leader may give some examples to help clarify the idea.

Making Captions

Goal: To encourage creative thinking.

Description: Tape pictures up on walls around the room. Have participants write a title, remark or caption for each picture. Allow people to mill about the room — like being at an exhibit or museum. Set and state a time limit. Give people a few reminders to let them know how much time is left. The leader then has the group sit and go over pictures one by one and talk about captions. What similar and different thoughts, ideas, feelings come up? How do these relate to various issues/points they are dealing with? How do individuals in the group tend to view things?

Materials: Photos from magazines, pictures of paintings. In order to reuse the photos/pictures, mount them on construction paper or thin foam board. Participants will need paper and pencils/pens for writing captions.

Setting: The leader can demonstrate by giving one example of a caption.

Music and Markers

Goals: To encourage expression. To facilitate group interaction. It may be used as an introduction to creative expression.

Description: Each participant has a piece of paper. The music begins and group members close their eyes. They may listen to the music as long as they wish. When each member feels like it, s/he may select a marker and make a mark on the paper with eyes opened or closed. When the music stops, words or other markings may be added. Those who wish to discuss any part of what they wrote or how the music makes them feel may do so. The process may be repeated with different music. After the exercise has been completed, members of the group hold their work in front of them and arrange themselves to form a "rainbow" of colors with the work they've done. The rainbow incorporates all colors and creates splendor that far surpasses the beauty of one color. The facilitator can congratulate the group for the diversity of its artistic expression and how it creates a rainbow of color and creativity.

Materials: Tape recorder or CD player; music without words; perhaps classical or quiet jazz; a large quantity of markers of as many colors as possible; paper.

Setting: Non-threatening activity; participants work individually as well as together. This is a good activity to use with clients who are functioning at a lower level, or with those who are having difficulty writing down words or thoughts. It will be up to the facilitator to decide how long the music should play. Any kind of music is acceptable as long as there are no words.

Alternate Forms of Poetry

These next three highly stylized forms of poetry may not be familiar to the group. Experimenting with any of them provides a good learning activity and an effective means of expressing thoughts and feelings.

Syntu

Goals: learn a new form of poetry, think creatively, be able to express emotions and feeling about others in writing.

Directions: Have clients pair up or form groups. Each client then tells the other member(s) of their group something really nice about themselves that s/he has refrained from saying during the previous seven weeks. Ask group to think about how they feel when they're giving a compliment and/or receiving one. After the compliment-giving is over, explain to clients that they may write a "syntu" about friendship. A syntu is a five-line poem written in the following form with one or two words to as line:

subject:	friends
descriptive word:	comforting
emotion felt by writer:	loving
descriptive word:	necessary
synonym for subject:	support system

Materials: Paper, crayons, pencils.

Setting: The leader should explain what a syntu is and read one example to the group.

Haiku

Goals: To be able to express emotions and feelings about others in writing. To think creatively.

Description: A haiku is a tightly structured three-line, 17 syllable verse form with an emphasis on images from nature and rhythms. Haiku are originally found in Japanese literature. They came about through the Japanese love of nature and beauty. Haiku attempt to evoke a feeling and an create an image with a minimum of words. Haiku evolved during the 14th century. The monks of the Zen sect of Buddhism adopted the form during the 15th century. One of the monks, Yamazaki Sakon (1465-1553) is known as the father of Haiku because he was the first poet to use the form separately from

the larger body of poetry in which it originally appeared. There are five important things to remember when creating a haiku.
1. It should provide a clear image.
2. It must come from the heart/be sincere.
3. It should not preach.
4. It must be a simple statement of what is.
5. It is usually associated with a season of the year.

The following example shows the structure of a haiku with the syllable count shown.

>   *1   2 3   4   5*
> *Hungrily searching*
>   *1   2   3   4   5 6   7*
> *Seagulls swirling overhead*
>   *1 2   3   4   5*
> *Rising with the wind*

Materials: pens/pencils, paper, examples of haiku, (optional) Japanese music, tape recorder.
Setting: The leader reads some examples of haiku and gives a brief background on its history.

Diamonte
Goals: To learn a new form of poetry and to think creatively. To be able to express emotions and feelings about other people, places or things in writing.
Description: A diamonte is a seven line poem with an ascending and descending number of words. The words form the shape of a diamond (*diamonte)* on the page.
- 1 noun (name of person, place or thing).
- 2 adjectives describing the first noun.
- 3 verbs that are actions of the first noun.
- 4 nouns (associated with the nouns at top and bottom).
- 3 verbs that are actions of the last noun.
- 2 adjectives describing last noun.
- 1 noun which is the opposite of the first noun.

Materials: Paper, crayons, pencils.

Setting: The leader should explain what a diamonte is and read one example to the group.

Inter-Being

If you are a poet, you will see clearly that there is a cloud floating in this sheet of paper. Without a cloud, there will be no rain; without rain, the trees cannot grow; and without trees we cannot make paper. The cloud is essential for the paper to exist. If the cloud is not here, the sheet of paper cannot be here either. So we can say that the cloud and the paper inter-are. "Inter-being" is a word that is not in the dictionary yet.

If we look into this sheet of paper even more deeply, we can see sunshine in it. If the sunshine is not there, the forest cannot grow. In fact, nothing can grow. Even we cannot grow without sunshine. And so we know that the sunshine is also in this sheet of paper. The paper and the sunshine inter-are. And if we continue to look we can see the logger who cut the tree and brought it to the mill to be transformed into paper. And we see the wheat. We know the logger cannot exist without his daily bread, and therefore the wheat that became his bread is also in this sheet of paper. Looking even more deeply, we can see we are in it too. This is not difficult to see, because when we look at a sheet of paper, the sheet of paper is part of our perception. Your mind is in here and mine is also. So we can say that everything is in here with this sheet of paper. You cannot point out one thing that is not here — time, space, the earth, the rain, the minerals in the soil, the sunshine, the cloud, the river, the heat. Everything co-exists with this sheet of paper. To be is to inter-be. You cannot just be by yourself alone. You have to inter-be with every other thing. This sheet of paper is, because everything else is.

— Thich Nhat Hanh: The Heart of Understanding

15

Meditation and Creative Visualization

The creative process seems to take place with greater ease when we are in a state of relaxed awareness. In this state we can be freed from our standard responses and beliefs and discover new images and ways of thinking.

There are situations which at first glance seem totally separated from the creative process, but which are actually conducive to creative reflection. Some are relaxing, such as taking a walk or daydreaming while others demand a person's full attention, such as meditation, writing, house cleaning or physical labor.

In order to reap the most benefit from the creative process, we should learn to relax and listen to our inner dialogue without judgment or censorship, to be an objective observer. The paradox is that when we're "trying to get an answer" this demand we put on ourselves defeats our purpose. What is creative may appear as an image, an idea that may seem to be almost wordless, a feeling, intuition, emotional response, an inspiration or insight. Welcome it, for its true value may not be revealed at once.

Write down with words, drawings, notations or symbols the thoughts and images that have come to mind. Although these messages emerge from deep within us, we are able to work with them once we allow them to be revealed to us.

Meditation

Meditation is any activity that keeps the attention pleasantly anchored in the present moment. Think of an activity that you really enjoy. I (Ann Nathan) am sitting here at the typewriter on a hot summer day. I'm sweating profusely and I fantasize for a moment. I approach a beautiful lake. I notice the trees, flowers and grass. The wind is warm as it blows over me. Now I wade into the lake and then dive in. I pause and enjoy my own sense of the cooling water. Ahh. For a moment the world stops. I am no longer concerned with books, bills, shopping, relationships or any other thoughts. I surrender to the immediate pleasure of the water. That's what enjoyment is. Surrender. Letting go of all the things pulling you out of the moment.

For once, the mind is not reading its list of things that must happen before we can be happy. It's not reciting the list of awful things that could happen to steal our happiness. It has taken a back seat to just being. This is the meditative state that elicits the relaxation response. It is peace.

The following exercise can be used to induce a meditative state.

Meditation Exercise
Choose a quiet spot where you will not be disturbed by other people or by the telephone.

Sit in a comfortable position, with back straight and arms and legs uncrossed, unless you choose to sit cross-legged on a floor cushion.

Close your eyes. This makes it easier to concentrate.

Relax your muscles sequentially from head to feet. This step helps to break the connection between stressful thoughts and a tense body. As you do this, breath slowly in and out. For now, just become aware of each part of your body in succession, letting go as much as you can with the out breath. Take a second now just to take a deep breath in. Let it go. Notice how your body relaxes as you let go. This is the good old sigh of relief. The pull of gravity is always present, encouraging us to let go, but if there is no awareness of being tense, there can't be any letting go. Notice your shoulders right now. Is there any room to let them down more, cooperating with gravity and your own out breath? Every out breath is an opportunity to let go. Starting with your forehead, become aware of tension as you breathe in. Let go of any obvious tension as you breathe out. Go through the rest of your body in this way, proceeding down through your eyes, jaws, neck, shoulders, arms, hands, chest, upper back, middle back and midriff, lower back, belly, pelvis, buttocks, thighs, calves and feet. This need only take a minute or two.

Become aware of your breathing, noticing how the breath goes in and out, without trying to control it in any way. You may notice that your breathing gets slower and shallower as the meditation progresses. This is due to the physiological effects of the relaxation response, the fact that your body requires less oxygen because your metabolism has slowed down.

Choose a focus word or phrase that evokes a sense of meaning that is important to you. This could be anything at all. If you cannot think of one, you might want to try a very old Sanskrit mantra, Ham Sah. (Ham means "I am" and Sah means "That.") Repeat your focus word silently in time to your breathing. In the case of Ham Sah, just listen to your breath, imagining that it sounds like "Ham" on the in breath and "Sah" on the out breath.

Don't worry about how you are doing. As soon as you start to worry about whether you are doing it right, you have shifted from meditation to anxiety. If you notice that tendency, try labeling it, saying to yourself "judging, judging." Then let go, coming back to the breath and the focus, which are your anchors in the shifting tides of the mind. Your mind will not stop for more than seconds at a time, if at all, so don't expect it to. What happens is that that part of yourself that can watch or witness the shenanigans of the mind is learning to flex its muscles. Each time you notice that you've drifted into thought, try labeling where you were. For instance, "thinking, thinking" or "anger, anger "or "judging, judging" and then let it go, getting back to the anchor. In this way, you begin to train your mind in awareness — the antidote to denial and mental unconsciousness. The awareness you develop in meditation will begin to carry over into life, affording you much more choice in how you respond and restoring your ability to enjoy life. The most common experience and complaint about meditation is "I can't stop my mind from wandering." That's fine. Don't try. Just practice bringing it back to concentration on the breath and focus whenever you notice it wandering.

Practice at least once a day for ten to twenty minutes. Remember that practice is indispensable to progress in anything you do. In meditation your goals are twofold. The session itself is the goal. In the true sense, the process is the product. Your main goal is to sit and do the meditation. Even if it seems that the only thing you're doing is chasing after your mind to tie it down again, remarkably, the relaxation response is still most likely occurring. Long before patients think they know "how to do it," they begin to notice that they are generally feeling more peaceful and their symptoms are beginning to improve. That, of course, *is* the second goal. Meditation does become easier and more deeply peaceful after repeated practice. If you can sit twice a day for ten to twenty minutes, so much the better. The preferred times are early morning, after a shower and exercise (if that is part of your regime) but before breakfast, or before dinner. The only times to avoid are when you're tired — simply because meditation is a concentration exercise and, if you're tired, you'll fall asleep—and just after a heavy meal, since the process of digestion makes people sluggish.

Creative Visualization

Creative visualization uses the imagination to help create what you want in your life. When you are visualizing, you use your imagination — your capacity to create images, emotions and thoughts in your mind — to create a vivid image of something you wish to make real in your life. You create and visit with this image regularly and continue until it becomes objective reality. This is not prayer, and you need not believe in a higher being. What is necessary is to want to expand your experience and understanding of life and be willing to try something new without being cynical or negative. Therapists have said that this technique deals with an image in a conscious way in order to challenge any possible unconscious reluctance to interact directly with the image.

What you want to make real could be cognitive, spiritual, physical or emotional or a combination of these elements. Examples include a new home, a home that is easier to keep clean, a new job, recognition for the job you're doing, a promotion, satisfaction at work, feeling calm and focused, being more calm and focused with specific people in your life, a complete, fulfilling relationship, grace under pressure — in general or in a specific situation, acceptance of a difficult reality or finally getting started on a creative endeavor. Other helpful areas on which to focus creative visualizations include:

Relationships
- conflict resolution
- showing and receiving affection
- loss and letting go
- commitment

Self-improvement
- being more patient
- test-taking
- accepting appearance
- stopping smoking

Health
- stress reduction
- eating and weight concerns
- peaceful, refreshing sleep
- recovery from illness or injury
- preparing for surgery or other treatment
- regaining strength after surgery or treatment
- medication — feeling it work
- talking to your body
- going to the dentist

Job and Career
- motivation to seek work
- feeling confident to call
- going on an interview
- asking for a raise
- giving birth or assisting in a birth
- changing careers
- handling conflict with co-workers

Affirmations

Affirmations are one of the most important, productive and life-changing ways to use creative visualization. An affirmation is a very strong, positive statement that something *is* the way we wish it to be, that it has happened. This adds another dimension to what you are imagining.

Many of us have an almost non-stop monologue (and sometimes conversation) going on in our minds. The mind talks to (some would say "at") itself in an endless commentary about all facets of our physical and emotional life. When we listen to ourselves, we become aware of how our mind works and often, how negative and self-critical it can be. For example, a person might catch his/her mind saying repeatedly, "This will never work," a thought that could affect the outcome of a situation. In other words, our inner monologue may follow set patterns and just becoming aware of what these patterns are can be very useful.

Affirmations, which are new and productive patterns, can be expressed in many ways. Some people prefer to say them aloud, while others prefer to say them silently, write them down, sing or chant them.

The following guidelines have proven helpful:
- Always word your affirmation as if it had already happened, now, in the present.
- Make it positive — what you want. Don't talk about what you do not want.
- Use your own words or take great care that what you say is exactly what you want, that it's just right for you.

Some examples of positive affirmations:
- I can do well in class.
- I can control my temper.
- I am able to be happy.
- I am a nice person.
- I can pass this test.

If we are able to forgive ourselves and others, if we can let go of disappointment, heartache, resentments and guilt, the tremendous blessing of emotional healing awaits us. It *is* within our grasp.

Often we feel that someone has taken something away from us: our faith in ourselves, a job, opportunity, love, money or optimism. We think we have lost our best selves to someone who has cheated us out of them, who has robbed us of our peace of mind.

The guidelines listed here can be very helpful in creating a visualization-affirmation process. You have a lot to lose, and it weighs you down more than the pounds you may struggle to lose on a diet.

Visualization and Affirmation of Forgiveness

Relax your body and mind. Follow relaxation techniques found in this book or elsewhere. Breathe deeply through your center which is just below your navel. Close your eyes.

Imagine a beautiful, peaceful setting which is calm and without distractions. You can imagine yourself walking, or swimming, as well as in a reclining position.

Visualize the person you have not forgiven. He or she is walking toward you. You see this person as a human being, like you, moving through life and trying to learn, as you are. If the usual negative thoughts begin to emerge, rewind the scene as if it were film or remove the person and start again until he or she can approach you without carrying negative feelings. You walk up to where the other person is standing and say something like, "I forgive you totally and you totally forgive me. All that is not harmonious between us disappears. I let go of all bad feelings I have towards you. We are both free now to pursue what is best about both of us." Remember, if these words do not suit you, make your own. After you've selected the words you want to use, if they begin to take on an air of insincerity, or of you're saying them through clenched teeth, stop and begin again.

If you feel that you lost something important because of this person, imagine the person giving you a box that has the name of what you feel has been lost. For example, "faith in men" or "trust in women" or "love" or "my security." Picture the person saying "I'm giving this back to you. This is yours, this is for you, your loss is over, now this has ended" or something that sounds right to you. Then imagine that the package begins to glow with a beautiful light, full of energy, and this becomes one with you.

Imagine that each of you begins to glow, you smile at each other and then either walk away, fly away or whatever seems appropriate to you. You go in different directions.

If you can't get to the end of the exercise — if you just can't let go — be aware of that. Sometimes you may have to continue to talk about it with yourself and others before you can get through the whole exercise.

Sometimes you may make it through the whole exercise but find later that you still have unresolved feelings. Continue to work on this exercise. Real progress is rarely achieved overnight. A better life awaits you, it's already yours, you need only claim it.

Sample Scripts

These sample scripts can be used and modified as required for individual situations.

Advisor
Allow yourself to totally relax your mind and body. When you feel yourself deeply relaxed, imagine a place that is beautiful and peaceful. It might be a quiet isolated beach, a lovely meadow on a spring afternoon, or a spectacular view from a mountain top. It might be a place where you have vacationed and where you re- member being very happy and relaxed.

When you feel yourself very comfortable in this beautiful place, look for the person whom you have come here to see. If you don't see that person at first, keep looking. When the figure appears, ask him/her to talk with you. Tell the person why you have come look- ing for him/her. Allow yourself to be with this person as comforta- bly as you would be with a friend in your own home.

When you feel comfortable and accepting of your adviser, ask him/her a question(s) that you have been wanting to ask. Then wait patiently for the answer. If an answer doesn't come immediately, ask your adviser how you can find the answer to your question.

Keep asking questions until you have the answer(s) you have sought. When your answers come, and you feel satisfied that they are what you sought, thank your adviser and tell him/her that you will return again to visit. Know that it is always within your reach.

Allow yourself to return here and feel good; to feel that you have found out what you wanted to know and have the ability to use the information you have received.

Remember the beautiful place and use the adviser within you.

Relaxing the Body
Close your eyes. Get comfortable, and concentrate on your breathing.

Pay careful attention to your breathing. Recognize how slow and deep breathing will help to induce relaxation. Exhale. Then take a deep breath in through your nose and blow it out through your mouth. Breathe from your abdomen; deeply and slowly.

As you concentrate on your breathing, focus your attention on an imaginary spot in the center of your forehead. Look at the spot as if you were trying to see it from inside your head.

You will begin to realize that your eyelids have become tense. Get a sense of how tense the eyelids can become as you stare at the spot so that you can compare this feeling with relaxation.

When your eyelids become strained and uncomfortable, let them drop.

Notice the feeling of relaxation that radiates all through and around your eyes. Allow that feeling of warmth and relaxation to move out to the temples and across the forehead.

Let the relaxation then radiate to your scalp, to the back of your head, to your ears, temples, cheeks, nose, to your mouth and chin.

As you feel the tension leave your face, relax your jaw muscles. Let your jaw open slightly, so all the tension can smoothly flow away.

Relax the muscles in your neck. As you do, let your head tip forward gently so your chin just about touches your chest.

Let this feeling of relaxation flow down into your shoulder and from there into the muscles of your arms and hands, then down your back, over to the front of the chest, on down to the abdomen, and then allow it to reach all the way down to the base of the spine.

Let the buttocks go completely loose and limp. Allow the warmth and relaxation to spread to the thighs, on down the legs, down to the ankles, and down through the feet to the tips of the toes.

Now you feel completely relaxed. Take a moment, starting from the top of your head and working down, to check to see if any part of you is not yet fully relaxed.

If you find any part of your body not fully relaxed, simply inhale a deep breath and send it into the area, bringing soothing, healing, relaxing, nourishing oxygen to comfort that area. As you exhale, imagine blowing out through your skin any tension, tightness or discomfort. By inhaling a breath into that area and exhaling right through the skin, you are able to replace tension in any part of your body with gentle relaxation.

When you find yourself quiet and fully relaxed, take a few moments to enjoy it.

Creative Visualization/Imagery Resources

Books

Achterberg, J. 1985. **Imagery in Healing: Shamanism and Modern Medicine.** Boston, MA: New Science Library/Shambala.
Provides in depth scientific underpinnings to the imagery techniques and provides a historical account of non-medical healing in the Western world.
Benson, H., MD. 1976. **The Relaxation Response.** New York, NY: Avon Books.
Dr. Benson is a pioneering researcher of the physiology of meditation and discovered it triggers a physiological reflex he calls the relaxation response.
Borysenko, J., Ph.D. 1987. **Minding the Body, Mending the Mind.** Reading, MA: Addison-Wesley.
A clear and useful book about self-healing by the former director of the Mind-Body Clinic at the New England Deaconess Hospital. Dr. Borysenko is a microbiologist, psychologist and yoga instructor.
Fanning, P. 1994. **Visualization for Change: Second Edition.** Oakland, CA: New Harbinger.
Rossman, M., MD. 1988. **Healing Yourself: A Step-By Step Program For Better Health Through Imagery.** New York, NY: An Institute For the Advancement Of Health Book. Walker & Co.

Tapes

Fanning, P. 1992. *Stress Reduction* (Audio Tape)
      Allergies and Asthma (Audio Tape)
      Treating Cancer (Audio Tape)
      Healing Injuries (Audio Tape)
      Curing Infectious Diseases (Audio Tape)
      Shyness (Audio Tape).
      Oakland, CA: New Harbinger.

Halpern, S. *Steve Halpern Tapes* (Audio Tape). Belmont, CA.
      The "Mozart of the New Age." Selection of relaxing music
      tapes with and without subliminal messages from reducing
      pain to increasing memory. Send for free catalogue.

Insight Publishing: Mill Valley, CA. Lecture tapes, tapes on im-
      agery, self-healing and related topics by prominent authori-
      ties in the field. Send for free catalogue.

Institute For The Advancement Of Human Behavior: Stanford,
      CA. Wide variety of tapes.

Kane, J. 1992. *Transforming Your Chronic Pain* (Audio Tape).
      Oakland, CA: New Harbinger.

Miller, E. MD. *The Source* (Audio Tape). Menlo Park, CA: Emmet
      Miller Tapes:
      High quality tapes from pain relief to surgery preparation
      and healing etc. Send for catalogue.

References

Adler, C. and G. Stanford, S. M. Adler. 1976. **We Are But a Moment's Sunlight: Understanding Death.** New York, NY: Pocket Books.

Avedon, E. 1974. **Therapeutic Recreation Service.** Englewood Cliffs, NJ: Prentice-Hall, Inc.

Bitcon, C. H. 1976. **Alike and Different: The Clinical and Educational Use of Orff Schulwerk.** Santa Ana, CA: Rosha Press.

Blatner, A. 1989. **Acting In: Practical Applications of Psychodramatic Methods.** New York, NY: Springer Publications.

Brammer, L. 1985. **The Helping Relationship: Process and Skills.** Englewood Cliffs, NJ: Prentice-Hall, Inc.

Bresler, E. 1981. "The Use of Poetry Therapy with Older People." *Aging*, Jan.-Feb. pp. 23-25.

Browne, S. E. and N. Stern. 1985. **With the Power of Each Breath**. Pittsburgh, PA: Cleis Press.

Burg, B. 1980, April. "Viewpoint: Bibliotherapy and Poetry Therapy." *Programming Trends in Therapeutic Recreation.* 1(2).

Corsini, R. 1966. **Role-playing as Psychotherapy: A Manual.** Hawthorne, NY: Aldine de Gruyter.

Coyle, C., W. B. Kinney, B. Riley and J. Shank. 1991. **Benefits of Therapeutic Recreation.** Ravensdale, WA: Idyll Arbor, Inc.

Csikszentmihalyi, M. 1996. **Creativity.** New York, NY: Harper Collins Publishers, Inc.

Deighton, L. C. (ed.) 1971. **The Encyclopedia of Education, Volume 7.** New York, NY: Macmillan Pub. Co.

Denny, J. 1972. "Techniques for Individual and Group Art Therapy." *American Journal of Art Therapy.* 2(3), 117-134.

Department of Recreation and Leisure Studies, San Jose State University. **Closing the Gap: An In-Service Training Guide for Mainstreaming Recreation and Leisure Services.** A Project of the Department of Recreation and Leisure Studies, San Jose

State University, San Jose, CA. 1983. Distributed by the Office of Special Education, US Department of Education.

Edwards, B. 1989. **Drawing on the Right Side of the Brain.** New York, NY: St. Martin's Press.

Emunah, R. 1994. **Acting for Real: Drama Therapy Process, Technique and Performance.** New York, NY: Brunner/Mazel Publisher.

Feder, B. and E. Feder. 1981. **The Expressive Art Therapies.** Englewood Cliffs, NJ: Prentice-Hall, Inc.

Gaston, E. T. 1968. **Music in Therapy.** New York, NY: Macmillan Co.

Gregson, B. 1982. **The Incredible Indoor Game Book: 160 Group Projects, Games and Activities.** Belmont, CA: Fearon Teachers' Aids.

Hackett, L. and R. Jenson. 1973. **Movement Exploration.** Palo Alto, CA: Peek Publications.

Kellogg, R. and S. O'Dell. 1967. **The Psychology of Children's Art: A Psychology Today Book.** San Diego, CA: CRM-Random House Publications.

Kübler-Ross, E. 1978. **To Live Until We Say Good-Bye.** Englewood Cliffs, NJ: Prentice-Hall, Inc.

Landgarten, H. 1981. **Clinical Art Therapy: A Comprehensive Guide.** New York, NY: Brunner/Mazel Publisher.

Leedy, J. 1969. **Poetry Therapy: The Use of Poetry in the Treatment of Emotional Disorders.** Philadelphia, PA: J. B. Lippincott Co.

Leveton, E. 1977. **Psychodrama for the Timid Clinician.** New York, NY: Springer Pub. Co.

Lorenz, K. 1963. **On Aggression.** New York, NY: Harcourt, Brace and World.

Luft, J. 1984. **Group Processes: An Introduction to Group Dynamics — Third Edition.** Mountain View, CA: Mayfield Publishers.

McNeely, D. 1987. **Touching: Body Therapy and Depth Psychology (Studies in Jungian Psychology No. 30).** Toronto, Ontario, Canada: Inner City Books.

McTwigan, M. and H. Post. 1973. **Clay Play: Learning Games for Children.** Englewood Cliffs, NJ: Prentice-Hall, Inc.

Maslow, A. H. 1968. **Toward a Psychology of Being.** New York, NY: John Wiley & Sons.

Maslow, A. H. 1987. **Motivation and Personality.** New York: Harpercollins College Division.

Moreno, J. L. 1985. **Psychodrama.** Boston, MA: Beacon House.

Peterson, C.A. 1976, April. "State of the Art Activity Analysis." In *Leisure Activity Participation and Handicapped Populations: Assessment of Research Needs,* NRPA and BEH.

Progoff, I. 1975. **At a Journal Workshop.** New York, NY: Dialogue House Library.

Rico, G. 1983. **Writing the Natural Way.** Los Angeles, CA: J. P. Tarcher, Inc.

Rubin, J. 1984. **The Art of Art Therapy.** New York, NY: Brunner/Mazel Publisher.

Spolin, V. 1983. **Improvisation for the Theater: A Handbook of Teaching and Directing — Revised Edition.** Evanston, IL: Northwestern University Press.

Striker, S. and E. Kimmel. 1987. **AntiColoring Book.** New York, NY: Holt, Rinehart and Winston.

The Older Adult Resource Center Newsletter, sponsored by the Peralta Community College District. Special issue on the creative works of older adults, Number 5, May/June 1980.

Ulman, E. 1996. **Art Therapy: In Theory and Practice**. Chicago, IL: Magnolia Street Publishers.

Valiant. G. E. 1977. **Adaptation to Life.** Boston, MA: Little, Brown.

Virshup, E. 1973. **Right Brain People in a Left Brain World.** Los Angeles, CA: Guild of Tutors Press.

Von Oech, R. 1993. **A Whack on the Side of the Head.** New York, NY: Warner Books.

Warren, B. 1984. **Using the Creative Arts in Therapy.** Cambridge, MA: Brookline Books.

Wilson, H. and C. Kneisl. 1996. **Psychiatric Nursing.** Menlo Park, CA: Addison Wesley Nursing Publications.

Winner, E. 1986. "Where Pelicans Kiss Seals." *Psychology Today.* 20(7) pp. 25-35.

Yablonsky, L. 1976. **Psychodrama.** New York, NY: Basic Books, Inc.

Yalom, I. 1975. **Theory and Practice of Group Psychotherapy.** New York, NY: Basic Books, Inc.

Index

activities
  clay, 111
  dance/movement, 217–23
  mask, 135–39
  movement exploration, 225–32
  music, 206–13
  painting and drawing, 108
  poetry and writing, 245–54
  psychodrama, 187–92
  role playing, 172–83
  separation, 74–77
  sociodrama, 183
  theater games, 162
  Viola Spolin's theater games, 155
  visual arts, 113–31
activity analysis, 5
affirmations, 264
aggregate interactions, 62
aggressive art materials, 107
almost pictures, 57
alternative communication, 3
art activity skills, 105
art in outline, 56
art materials, 94, 106
  aggressive, 107
  compulsive, 106
  expressive, 107
  regressive, 106
art space, 93

arthritis, 100
artist, 32
artistic skills
  development, 54
attention span deficits, 101
catharsis, 7
ceremonies for change, 77
checklist for groups, 83
child and design, 56
clay activities, 111
clown safety, 197
clowning, 193–202
compensatory techniques, 98
compulsive art materials, 106
crafts, 104
creative arts
  benefits, 2–5
  effectiveness, 6
creative person, 10
creative process, 14
creative thinking, 12
creative traits, 10
creative visualization. *See* meditation and creative visualization
creative writing, 236
creativity
  blocks to, 17
  definition, 10
  elements of, 9–25
  enhancing, 19

hindering, 23
rediscovering, 10
teaching, 18
dance/movement, 215–33
 goals, 215
dance/movement activities,
 217–23
developmental stages, 41
disabilities
 compensating for, 98
double (in role playing), 174
drama therapy, 171–92
 psychodrama, 184–92
 role playing, 171–83
 sociodrama, 183–84
drama therapy groups, 145–
 49
drawing, 107
drawing activities, 108
drawing people, 56
enhancing participation, 87
enjoyment, 15
evaluation, 86
expansiveness, 2
expressive art materials, 107
external communication, 3
facilitating, 28
fears about creativity, 19
fine arts, 104
flow experience, 15
freedom, 2
funding, 90
goals, 81
group members, 84
groups

checklist, 83
clowning, 193–202
dance/movement, 215–33
drama therapy, 145–49,
 171–92
dynamics, 39
enhancing creativity, 19
goals, 81
helping relationship, 68
hindering creativity, 23
individuals in, 39–78
interaction patterns, 61
logistics, 82
meditation and creative
 visualization, 259–71
movement exploration,
 215–33
music therapy, 203–13
planning, 79–101
poetry and writing, 235–58
psychological
 development, 66
separation, 74–77
stages of psychological
 development, 61
theater games and
 improvisation, 151–70
healing, 4
helping relationship, 39, 68
improvisation, 152. *See also*
 theater games and
 improvisation
individuals
 in therapy groups, 39–78
interactions

aggregate, 62
inter-group, 65
inter-individual, 63
internal, 61
intra-group, 65
multi-lateral, 64
object-oriented, 61
unilateral, 64
inter-group interactions, 65
inter-individual interactions, 63
internal communication, 2
internal interaction, 61
interpersonal relations, 4
intra-group interactions, 65
Johari windows, 58
leader responsibilities, 83
left-brain thinking, 12
leisure, 3
life situations (for role playing), 176
lifestyle considerations, 89
limited vision, 99
logistics, 82
mandalas, 56
mask activities, 135–39
masks, 133–43
creating, 134, 139
papier mache, 140
plaster gauze, 142
therapeutic, 134
Maslow, Abraham, 4
meditation, 260
meditation and creative visualization, 259–71

movement exploration, 215–33
movement exploration goals, 224–32
movement exploration activities, 225–32
multicultural considerations, 89
multi-lateral interactions, 64
music
Orff Schulwerk, 206
Orff Schulwerk rondos, 206–11
music activities, 206–13
music therapy, 203–13
object-oriented interactions, 61
Orff Schulwerk
rondos, 206–11
Orff, Carl, 206
painting, 108
painting activities, 108
papier mache masks, 140
paradoxical traits, 12
participation enhancing, 87
pictures, 57
planning, 79–101
plaster gauze masks, 142
poetry and writing, 235–58
poetry and writing activities, 245–54
poetry therapy, 236
preparation, 84
program justification, 79

psychodrama, 184–92
  elements of, 185
  techniques, 187–92
psychodrama activities, 187–92
regressive art materials, 106
resources and funding, 93
resources and funding, 90
respiratory problems, 100
right-brain thinking, 3, 12
role playing, 171–83
  guidelines, 172
  life situations, 176
rondos. *See* Orff Schulwerk
scribbles and scribbling, 55
scripts, 267
secrets of shape, 56
self-worth, 4
sensitive skin, 100
separation activities, 74–77
session planning, 85
sharing, 15
skills for art activities, 105
skin sensitivity, 100
sociodrama, 183–84
space considerations, 80
Spolin, Viola, 153

spontaneity, 153
stages of development, 41
standards, 84
tactile arts, 103–31
teaching, 31
theater game activities, 162
theater games, 152
theater games and
  improvisation, 151–70
therapeutic art, 104
therapist, 34
  roles, 27–37
therapy groups. *See* groups
unilateral interactions, 64
Viola Spolin's theater games,
  155
vision
  limited, 99
visual arts, 103–31
visual arts activities, 113–31
visual arts experiences, 104
visual arts groups
  planning, 93
whole arm drawing, 55
writing. *See* poetry and
  writing

About the Authors

Ann Argé Nathan was a vibrant woman who lived her life fully for 47 years. In her short life she accomplished much, experiencing life to the fullest and leaving a mark on the lives of everyone she touched. A Recreational Therapist, educator, consultant and author, Ann received degrees from, and taught at both San José and San Francisco State Universities. She practiced at Langley Porter Neuropsychiatric Institute at the University of California, San Francisco, and other clinical settings.

Raised in Berkeley, California, Ann was deeply influenced in her life's activities by her parents, Ed and Harriet Nathan. They instilled in her a love for learning, social activism and helping others. Recreational Therapy became her lifelong vocation and she brought a passion to her practice and her teaching that motivated clients and students alike. While teaching at San Francisco State University, Ann was the Coordinator for Therapeutic Recreation along with Clinical Supervisor for internships.

Ann served as a trainer/consultant on more than a score of projects throughout Northern California, including recovery services for the developmentally disabled and "at risk" youth and families. She was a co-therapist in an eating disorders group. She worked with clients from six months of age to ninety nine years of age in her career. Ann received numerous grants and awards for her work, including:

California Parks and Recreation Therapeutic Recreation Section *Play Award* (1986)

Meritorious Performance and Professional Promise Award, San Francisco State University (1987)

Outstanding Service Award, San Francisco State University Department of Recreation and Leisure Studies (1990)

California Parks and Recreation Therapeutic Recreation Section *Outstanding Educator Award* (1991)

Outstanding Teacher Award, San Francisco State University Department of Recreation and Leisure Studies (1993)

Ann died of breast cancer on January 8, 1995. Her work and her love of students will be remembered for many years to come. The Ann Argé Nathan Spirit Scholarship Award continues to honor her love of teaching by presenting three or four students whose studies have a special emphasis in therapeutic recreation with a scholarship award yearly during the California Parks and Recreation Convention.

Suzanne Mirviss has a Master's Degree in Recreation with Emphasis in Therapeutic Recreation from San Francisco State University. She has taught courses in the Recreation and Leisure Studies Department at both San José State and San Francisco State Universities. For over twenty years she has worked with many groups and is currently employed at the San Francisco VA Medical Center as an Art Consultant in the Psychiatric Day Treatment Center.

Ms. Mirviss received her training in drawing and painting from the San Francisco Academy of Art. She is devoted to the creative arts, volunteering in her community and local schools to support children's art expression. Ms. Mirviss is primarily a watercolor painter but also enjoys working with fused glass, enameling and jewelry. Ms. Mirviss lives in Marin County, California with her husband, two children and assorted family pets.

CPSIA information can be obtained at www.ICGtesting.com
Printed in the USA
BVOW07s1438291213

340329BV00002B/133/P